Current Issues in Nurse Prescribing

© 2001
Greenwich Medical Media Limited
137 Euston Road
London
NW1 2AA

ISBN 1-84110-063-3

First published 2001

A catalogue record for this book is available from the British Library.

Visit our website at:
www.greenwich-medical.co.uk

Distributed worldwide by Plymbridge Distributors Ltd

Typeset by Phoenix Photosetting, Chatham, Kent

Printed by Alden Press

Current Issues in Nurse Prescribing

Molly Courtenay

PhD, MSc, BSc, RGN, RNT, Cert Ed

Independent Consultant and Honorary Visiting Fellow
Department of Professional Education in Community Studies
The University of Reading

CONTENTS

Contributors   vii

Preface   vii

Chapter 1

The development of nurse prescribing: an overview   1
Molly Courtenay

Chapter 2

Legal and professional accountability for nurse prescribing   9
Breda Gibson

Chapter 3

Ethical issues in nurse prescribing   25
Paul Cain

Chapter 4

Clinical diagnosis and management for the nurse prescriber   39
Chris Derrett

Chapter 5

Current issues in nurse prescribing: a pharmacist's perspective   69
Beth Taylor and Laraine Clarke

Chapter 6

Nurse prescribing: an evaluation of an implementation programme within one health authority and two community healthcare trusts 89
Cynthia Thornton

Index 107

CONTRIBUTORS

Catherine Blowers RGN DN
Nurse Prescribing Project Nurse
West Berkshire PCS NHS Trust
Prospect Park Hospital
Reading, UK

Paul Cain MAOxon MA Dip Phil(Healthcare)
Dept. of Professional Education in Community Studies
The University of Reading
Reading, UK

Laraine Clark BPharm MSc MRPharmS
Prescribing Adviser
Canterbury and Coastal PCG
Chestfield Medical Centre
Whitstable, Kent

Molly Courtenay PhD MSc BSc RGN RNT Cert Ed
Independent Consultant and Honorary Visiting Fellow
Department of Professional Education in Community Studies
The University of Reading, UK

Christopher Derrett GP BSc Mphil MBBS MRCGP DRCOG DCH
Senior Lecturer
Dept. of General Practice and Primary Care
St Bartholomew's & The Royal London
School of Medicine & Dentistry
London, UK

Breda Gibson RGN DipN PGCEA RNT BA MA Dip HealthCare Law
Training and Development Consultant
South Ferring
Worthing, Uk

Mary Mullix RGN RSCN BA (Hons) MSc
Nurse Prescribing Project Nurse
Primary Care Services
St Mark's Hospital
Maidenhead, UK

Beth Taylor BSc MRPSGB
Pharmacy Manager
Community Health South London NHS Trust
Elizabeth Blackwell House
New Cross
London, UK

Cynthia Thornton MSc RGN DN PWT PGCEA DNT
Dept. of Professional Education in Community Studies
The University of Reading
Reading, UK

PREFACE

The introduction of nurse prescribing has meant that nurses have had to acquire new knowledge in a number of fields including ethics, law and Pharmacology. Furthermore, this knowledge has had to be applied to the many issues surrounding prescribing in the practice setting. As prescribing is a new area in which nurses have expanded their practice, there are currently few books available that provide prescribers with information to help them in this role. It is hoped that the information provided in this book will help to fill this gap.

Chapter 1 provides a general overview of the development of nurse prescribing and describes the current education and training available for prescribers. Chapters 2 and 3 describe the legal and ethical frameworks within which prescribers must practise. Practice scenarios are used to illustrate the application of this knowledge. Chapter 4 describes the clinical diagnosis and treatment management of a number of conditions for which nurses are involved in prescribing. Nurse prescribing from a pharmacist's perspective is presented in Chapter 5. Topics discussed include: how pharmacists can support nurse prescribers, sources of drug information, prescribing and group protocols, bulk purchasing, the development of prescribing guidelines and formularies, prescribing budgets and the use of prescription analysis and cost (PACT) reports. Finally, Chapter 6 provides a critical account of the implementation of nurse prescribing within one health authority and two adjoining community healthcare trusts. Issues that arose in relation to both education and practice are presented.

Molly Courtenay
Independent Consultant and Honorary
Visiting Fellow
Department of Professional Education
in Community Studies
The University of Reading
November, 2000

THE DEVELOPMENT OF NURSE PRESCRIBING: AN OVERVIEW

In 1986, recommendations were made for nurses to take on the role of prescribing. The Cumberlege Report *Neighbourhood Nursing: A Focus for Care* Department of Health and Social Security (DHSS, 1986) examined the care given to clients in their homes by district nurses (DNs) and health visitors (HVs). It was identified that some very complicated procedures had arisen around prescribing in the community and that nurses were wasting their time requesting prescriptions from the general practitioner (GP) for such items as wound dressings and ointments. The report suggested that patient care could be improved and resources used more effectively if community nurses were able to prescribe, as part of their everyday nursing practice, from a limited list of items and simple agents agreed by the DHSS.

Following the publication of this report, the recommendations for prescribing and its implications were examined. An advisory group was set up by the Department of Health (DoH) to examine nurse prescribing (Crown Report, DoH, 1989). Dr June Crown was the chair of this group. A number of recommendations were made involving the categories of items which nurses might prescribe, together with the circumstances under which they might be prescribed. It was recommended that:

'Suitably qualified nurses working in the community should be able, in clearly defined circumstances, to prescribe from a limited list of items and to adjust the timing and dosage of medicines within a set protocol.' (DoH, 1989)

The Crown Report identified several groups of patients that would benefit from nurse prescribing. These patients included: patients with a catheter or a stoma, patients suffering with postoperative wounds and homeless families not registered with a GP. The Report also suggested that a number of other benefits would occur as a result of nurses adopting the role of prescriber. As well as improved patient care, this included improved use of both patients' and nurses' time and improved communication between team members arising as a result of a clarification of professional responsibilities (DoH, 1989).

An empirical study commissioned by the DoH and undertaken prior to nurse prescribing was carried out by Touche Ross (DoH, 1991). This work aimed to identify the benefits and costs of nurse prescribing. Research methods involved questionnaires and interviews. It was evident from this study that there was widespread support for the 'principles of nurse prescribing'. It was forecast that nurses, GPs and patients would experience small weekly time savings if nurse prescribing was introduced. Another anticipated benefit was speedier access to products.

During 1992, the primary legislation permitting nurses to prescribe a limited range of drugs was passed (*Medicinal Products: Prescription by Nurses etc. Act 1992*). The necessary amendments were made to this Act in 1994 and a revised list of products available to the nurse prescriber was published in the Nurse Prescribers' Formulary (NPF) (Box 1.1). During this period, guidelines were issued to the DoH from the United Kingdom Central Council for Nursing, Midwifery, and Health Visiting (UKCC) and national boards with regard to the education that would be necessary to enable nurses to prescribe.

In 1994, eight demonstration sites were set up in England for nurse prescribing. Nurses working in these sites attended either the nurse-prescribing programme at the North East Surrey College of Technology or Manchester Metropolitan University, for the taught component of the nurse-prescribing programme (Mode 1 students).

Evaluation of pilot schemes has revealed a number of issues. A study by Luker *et al* (1997) identified from patient data that in some instances, patients chose to see a nurse as opposed to their GP. In some cases, the reason given for this was convenience. However, a number of patients

---

Box 1.1 – Items in the NPF English National Board (ENB, 1998)

- Laxatives

- Analgesics

- Local anaesthetics

- Drugs for the mouth

- Removal of ear wax

- Drugs for threadworm

- Drugs for scabies and head lice

- Skin preparations

- Disinfection and cleansing

- Wound management products

- Elastic hosiery

- Urinary catheters and appliances

- Stoma care products

- Appliances and reagents for diabetes

- Fertility and gynaecological products

---

considered nurses to have more expertise in certain clinical areas, e.g. wound care, and therefore sought their advice. It was also identified that, compared to the GP, nurses were found to be easier to talk to. Data collected from nurses illuminated that on the whole they enjoyed the experience of prescribing. There were both savings in time and increased job satisfaction. Nurses were also made more aware of the cost of items included in the NPF. Although anxieties were expressed about writing the first prescription, these anxieties disappeared once practitioners had settled in to their new role of prescriber. Some nurses in the study expressed concerns involving prescribing in conditions where a medical diagnosis was needed. This mainly involved laxatives, enemas and adult analgesia.

A further evaluation study (Blenkinsopp *et al*, 1998) involved the collection of data from nurse prescribers in two pilot sites (Walsall and Wigan). It was found that although the nurse-prescribing training programme was generally well received, it needed to be strengthened in the areas of pharmacology, choice of preparation to be prescribed and financial aspects of prescribing. It was also recommended that the taught component of the programme would benefit from an increased focus on case studies in order to maximise the application of learning to practice. These findings were confirmed and expanded in the second part of this study (Blenkinsopp and Savage, 1999) which also identified that there is a need for nurse prescribers to have further information on the use of Prescription Analysis and Cost Trends (PACT) reports in the self-monitoring of performance.

An extension of the pilot prescribing scheme took place in 1996 at Bolton, prior to its national roll-out. Over 100 nurses participated. Following evaluation, prescribing was expanded to one community trust in each region of England and two in Scotland.

The funding for full national implementation of nurse prescribing was promised by the government in 1998 by former Health Secretary Frank Dobson at the Royal College of Nursing (RCN) conference in April. It is anticipated that by the year 2001, approximately 20,000 DNs and HVs will be qualified prescribers. Additionally, postregistration programmes for DNs and HVs now include the necessary educational component qualifying nurses to prescribe (Mode 2 students).

A report on the supply and administration of medicines under group protocols was published in 1998 (DoH, 1998) and a further report by Crown, which reviewed the prescribing, supply and administration of medicines, was published in 1999. This review recommended that prescribing authority should be extended to other groups of professionals with training and expertise in specialised areas. A possible example that was given by the report was family planning nurses. The review team recommended that application for prescribing authority should be submitted to an advisory committee – the New Prescribers Advisory Committee. The role of this committee would be to assess applications from 'independent' and 'dependent' prescribers. Independent prescribers would be responsible for the assessment of patients with undiagnosed conditions and make decisions regarding their clinical management and prescribing. A dependent prescriber would be responsible for the continuing care of patients previously clinically assessed by an independent prescriber. This might include prescribing. However, prescribing by dependent prescribers would be informed by clinical guidelines and might involve adjusting the dose of medication or repeat prescriptions.

The government decided to take forward the recommendations of the review of prescribing in March 2000, with a view to having new regulations in place by July 2000. Health Minister Philip Hunt said:

> *'At present, highly skilled nurses are prevented from prescribing for common conditions because prescribing has always been seen as the traditional role of the hospital doctor or GP.*
>
> *That in turn has meant that hospital doctors' time is being taken up with tasks that could and should be performed by nurses and other health professionals.'*

It was envisaged that independent prescribing authority would initially be granted to specialist nurses. Following evaluation, independent status would then be extended to include other health professionals.

At the time of publication of this book, the governments NHS Plan (DoH 2000) suggests that both the range of medicines that can be prescribed by nurses and the number of nurses with prescribing powers will be extended. However, further clarification is waited. Patient Group Directions (PGDs) (see Chapter 5) and their role is enabling nurses to supply and administer medicines according to protocols is also highlighted in this document.

EDUCATION AND TRAINING FOR NURSE PRESCRIBERS

A number of criteria laid down by the Medicinal Products: Prescription by Nurses Act 1992, and subordinate legislation under the Act, identify those individuals able to prescribe from the NPF. At the time of publication of this book, in order to prescribe, the nurse must fulfil all the following criteria.

- She/he must be a first-level registered nurse with a DN or HV qualification or the respective recordable qualifications at specialist practice level

- She/he must work within a primary healthcare setting

- She/he must have successfully completed the nurse prescribers' programme

- She/he must be identified by the UKCC as a nurse prescriber

- She/he must be authorised/required by their employer to prescribe.

The nurse-prescribing course (Mode 1 students) is a two-part integrated programme of education and training. It comprises:

- an open learning pack which consists of distance learning material and acts as a bridge leading from the learner's current experience into the taught component

- a 15-hour taught component, which builds on the knowledge provided in the open learning pack.

The pack is divided into a number of sections. The areas covered include the following.

- The history and development of nurse prescribing

- Accountability

- Prescribing safely and effectively

- Ethical issues

- Prescribing in a team context

- Administrative arrangements

- Evaluating effectiveness (ENB, 1998).

Each section of the pack comprises a number of learning outcomes, a list of suggested readings and a number of activities. Learners are required to assess themselves as they work through the material. Students registered on the programme are provided with the pack and usually given half a study day, which introduces them to the course, 4–6 weeks before the start of the taught component. It was initially suggested that the distance learning material would take 10–12 hours study time. However, evaluation has shown that 20–25 hours is a more realistic allocation of time (Blenkinsopp et al, 1998).

The taught component of the programme involves 15 hours of study and runs over a two-week period. During this element, the areas covered in the open learning pack are further developed. Students attend lectures on three days and are then formally assessed. The assessment covers material from the open learning pack and the taught component of the course. Short answer questions and multiple choice questions combined with case studies, which students are asked to discuss, are typical assessment methods used. On passing the exam, nurses become registered nurse prescribers and are able to prescribe from the NPF.

CONCLUSION

Although it has been recommended that further evaluation should take place regarding economical evidence, nurse prescribing has been considered a success by patients, nurses, doctors and other professionals (Luker *et al*, 1997). The development of nurse prescribing has been slow. It has been under consideration by the government since 1986 and to date, prescribing has only been extended to nurses holding a HV or DN qualification. It was not until March 2000 that the government decided to take forward the recommendations of the review of prescribing and extend prescribing rights to other nursing groups. However, clarification is still awaited.

Before the extension of nurse prescribing can take place, there needs to be a review of pre- and postregistration nurse education. Appropriate input from the life sciences, i.e. anatomy, physiology, pharmacology, needs to be included in nurse education programmes. If nurse prescribers are to be accountable for their prescribing decisions, they must be equipped with the knowledge and skills to inform them about patient diagnosis, illness and prescribing treatment. It is important that nurse prescribing contributes to improving patient care and that every effort is made to ensure that patient safety remains a priority.

Nurse prescribing should not be viewed as a means of dealing with increasing medical workloads, nor as a means by which doctors are able to delegate undervalued tasks to nurses. Therefore, training and educational needs must be met with the appropriate resources and funding. This will ensure that nurses feel secure in their prescribing role and confident that they are acting within their level of clinical competence.

Nurse prescribing will have a direct impact on the role of the nurse. It will enable nurses to adopt a more holistic approach to patient care and should promote cohesiveness within the primary healthcare team. Most importantly, the flexibility of nurse prescribing will enable patient care to become more tailored to the needs of the individual. However, as nurses increase their responsibilities in other areas of care and undertake activities that were once viewed as the domain of medical staff, some essential nursing activities will inevitably be delegated to unregistered staff. This will undoubtedly affect future professional relationships and boundaries.

References

Blenkinsopp, A. & Savage, I. (1999). *Nurse Prescribing Evaluation (2): Continuing Development Needs.* Keele University: Department of Medicines Management.

Blenkinsopp, A., Grime, J., Pollock, K., Boardman, H. (1998). *Nurse Prescribing Evaluation (1): The Initial Training Programme and Implementation.* Keele University: Department of Medicines Management.

Department of Health (1989). *Report of the Advisory Group on Nurse Prescribing* (Crown Report). London: Department of Health.

Department of Health (1991). *Nurse Prescribing Final Report: A Cost Benefit Study* (Touche Ross Report) (unpublished). London: Department of Health.

Department of Health (1998). *Supply and Administration of Medicines under Group Protocols.* London: Department of Health.

Department of Health (1999). *Review of Prescribing, Supply and Administration of Medicines* (Crown Report). London: Department of Health.

Department of Health 2000. *The NAS Plan. A Plan for Investment. A Plan for Reform.* London: Dept. of Health.

Department of Health and Social Security (1986). *Neighbourhood Nursing: A Focus for Care* (Cumberlege Report). London: HMSO.

English National Board for Nursing, Midwifery and Health Visiting (1998*). Nurse Prescribing Open Learning Pack.* Milton Keynes: Learning Materials Design.

Luker, K.A., Austin, L., Hogg, C. (1997). *Evaluation of Nurse Prescribing: Final Report and Executive Summary.* Liverpool: University of Liverpool.

United Kingdom Central Council for Nursing, Midwifery and health Visiting (1994). *The Future of Professional Practice – The Council's Standard for Education and Practice Following Registration.* London: UKCC.

Acknowledgement

The author gratefully acknowledges the permission of *The British Journal of Community Nursing* to reproduce in this chapter some material from an article previously published in the journal (Volume 5, Number 3: March 2000: pages 122-125).

2

LEGAL AND PROFESSIONAL ACCOUNTABILITY FOR NURSE PRESCRIBING

THE LEGAL FRAMEWORK FOR NURSE PRESCRIBING

This chapter aims to explain the legal framework of nurse prescribing in order to increase awareness of and reflection on the legal background of nurse prescribing and the implications for personal accountability. Frequent reflection on practice is an implicit element in the United Kingdom Central Council (UKCC) *Scope of Professional Practice* (UKCC, 1992a). For nurse prescribers, this reflection will encompass all aspects of their new role and in particular their legal and professional duty of care for ensuring safe practice. This in turn requires the nurse to assess where potential breaches of duty may occur in prescribing and to take appropriate steps to minimise risks to patients. Failure to do so may make the nurse professionally and legally vulnerable in any allegation of negligence. Therefore, a basic knowledge of the law of negligence is essential for nurses prescribers practising in an increasingly litigious society. It is certainly the case that ignorance (of the law) is no defence.

The UKCC makes it clear that each nurse is personally accountable for actions taken and it is also evident that the law imposes the same standards of care on those in a trainee or inexperienced capacity. This may include nurses taking on new roles such as prescribing. In **Nettleship v Weston (1971)** cited in Tingle and Cribb (1995), it was held that 'a learner driver would be liable in negligence if he failed to drive as well as a reasonably competent driver'.

This chapter examines:

- the background to nurse prescribing
- relevant legislation
- the law of negligence
- areas of potential breaches of care in prescribing.

THE BACKGROUND TO NURSE PRESCRIBING

Healthcare practice does not exist in a vacuum; it occurs within the legal frameworks created by society. Just as society itself is constantly changing, so too does the law in order to reflect the needs of society. Within this context, nursing developments may require the drafting of new legislation or the amendment of existing legislation to ensure that nursing practice is founded on sound professional principles within a legal framework. The implementation of nurse prescribing required new legislation in the form of the *Medicinal products: Prescription by Nurses etc Act 1992*. In addition, amendments to the *Medicines Act 1968* and the *Pharmaceutical Services Regulations 1994* were necessary before nurses could legally prescribe.

Amendments to existing legislation

The Medicines Act 1968 governs the prescription, supply and storage of medicines. Under this Act, it is unlawful for anyone other than an 'appropriate practitioner' to prescribe drugs. Doctors, dentists, veterinary surgeons and veterinary practitioners are the appropriate practitioners defined in the Act. Section 58 of this Act was amended to include 'registered nurses, midwives and health visitors' in the list of appropriate practitioners.

The *Pharmaceutical Services Regulations 1994* were also amended to allow pharmacists to dispense from prescriptions written by nurses.

THE MEDICINAL PRODUCTS: PRESCRIPTION BY NURSES ETC ACT 1992

The Act permits appropriately qualified nurses to prescribe from a list contained in the Nurse Prescriber's Formulary (NPF), a subsection of the British National Formulary. The NPF contains items such as analgesics, laxatives, skin treatments, dressings, etc. (see Box 1.1).

Although this Act was passed in 1992, the necessary secondary legislation Medicinal Products; Prescription by Nurses etc Act 1992 (Commencement No 1) Order did not come into effect until 1994. An Order is a legislative document that enables the powers in an Act to be implemented and in addition, gives the legal definitions of the terms used within the Act. This Order specified the conditions which would have to be met before a nurse could prescribe and Section 2 states that an appropriate practitioner who is permitted to prescribe is a nurse:

- registered in Parts 1 or 12 of the UKCC Register a Registered General Nurse (RGN) who holds a current district nurse qualification and is a district nurse
- registered in Part 10 of the UKCC Register (a midwife)
- registered in Part 11 of the UKCC Register (a health visitor).

In addition, the authority to prescribe is limited to nurses who are employed by a district health authority or an NHS trust and who have completed the necessary educational preparation approved by a national board to the UKCC's standards.

The conditions specified in the legislation exclude nurses working in non-community settings. It could be argued that this is discriminatory and undermines not only the UKCC *Scope of Professional Practice* (UKCC, 1992b), but the work undertaken by many clinical nurse specialists.

This exclusion was reviewed in *the Review of Prescribing, Supply and Administration of Medicines Report* Department of Health (DoH 1999*)*, the recommendations of which were accepted by the government in March 2000. The report recommended that nurse prescribing be extended in the future to include nurses 'beyond currently authorised prescribers' and to allow prescribing by other healthcare professionals registered with a recognised regulatory body.

The report recommends the creation of two types of prescribers, 'independent' and 'dependent' prescribers, and the establishment of a New

---

Box 2.1 – The existing and new legislation required for nurse prescribing

- Medicines Act 1968

- Pharmaceutical Services Regulations 1994

- Medicinal Products; Prescription by Nurses etc Act 1992

Prescribers' Advisory Committee (NPAC) (see Chapter 1). It is not yet clear who will be empowered to be independent or dependent prescribers, nor is it clear what they will be permitted to prescribe. It is hoped that further consultations with appropriate professional groups will address these issues and the secondary legislation needed to establish this and to expand nurse prescribing is expected to be in place by 2001.

THE LAW OF NEGLIGENCE

The following explores Nurse Prescribing in relation to the law of negligence and includes:

- definition of negligence

- the duty of care in prescribing

- professional and legal definitions of standards of care

- potential breaches of duty of care prescribing.

Definition of negligence

In *Blyth v Birmingham Water Works (1856)* negligence was defined as 'the omission to do something which a reasonable man, guided upon these conditions which ordinarily regulate the conduct of human affairs would do or to do something which a prudent and reasonable man would not do'.

Duty of care

In law, NHS-employed doctors or nurses owe their patients a duty of care. This duty entails taking care and practising to a standard which will ensure that, as far as is reasonably practicable, patients are not caused harm or damage. If, however, this duty of care is breached and the patient can prove that any subsequent harm or damage is due to the breach, then they will have a right to sue for negligence. All three elements have to be proven, i.e. that a duty of care existed, that the duty was breached and that subsequent harm or damage was directly related to a breach of the duty of care. Nurses need to be aware of the nature of the duty of care they owe to patients.

The legal definition of duty of care was defined in **Donoghue v Stevenson (1932)** and is cited by Dimond (1995). The case involved a manufacturer being held liable for the existence of the decomposed remains of a snail found in one of its beer bottles. In this case, Lord Atkin stated that 'You must take reasonable care to avoid acts or omissions which you can reasonably foresee would be likely to injure your neighbour'. He defined 'neighbour' as '… Persons who are so closely and directly affected by my act that I ought reasonably to have them in contemplation as being so affected when I am directing my mind to the acts or omissions which are called in question'. It is evident from this definition that patients come into the category of 'neighbours' as far as nurses are concerned, i.e. persons to whom a duty of care is owed. The legal definition of duty of care is an integral part of the UKCC *Code of Professional Conduct* (UKCC, 1992b), which is not in itself a legal document but does affirm the principles of professional accountability. Nurses are accountable to the patient, the public, the profession and the employer. The nature of a nurse's legal duty of care to patients lies in their professional accountability for ensuring that patients are protected, have been given relevant and sufficient information before consenting to treatment and that they receive safe, quality care. Tingle (1990) states that 'However accountability is defined, and whatever the value of ethical codes, it is important to remember that the courts are the final venue for the resolution of disputes in medicine and nursing'.

In accepting new and expanded roles, nurses must be clear about their accountability and responsibility to determine whether their skills are relevant and up to date. They should also fully understand the nature of the tasks/responsibilities assigned to them. Additionally, Rieu (1994) stated that nurses must consider their competency before undertaking activities considered to be doctor's duties. This is particularly relevant to nurses undertaking prescribing responsibilities. It is clear from the *Scope of Professional Practice* (UKCC, 1992b) that nurses have a duty to acknowledge any limits of personal knowledge and skills and should not undertake activities which are outside their present level of competence. The nurse should compile a personal development plan to gain the required competence. Nurses should also determine the means by which the new skills are acquired and updated, in order to lessen the risk of breaches of duty of care.

Professional and legal standards of care

Any examination of alleged breaches of duty of care in prescribing will involve a comparison with accepted standards. The *Scope of Professional Practice* document states the broad principles for standards of professional practice. The law expects standards which do not result in patient harm and which are defined in terms of compatibility with other practitioners operating at that level of care. The standard of care was stated by McNair (cited in Kennedy and Grubb, 1989) as 'the standard of the ordinary skilled man exercising and professing to have that special skill'. The leading case for assessing the standard is ***Bolam vs Friern Barnet Hospital Management Committee (1957)*** which established the so-called 'Bolam principle' or 'test'. This is that 'A doctor is not negligent if he acts in accordance with a practice accepted at the time as proper by a responsible body of medical opinion'. It is evident that this principle can also be applied to nursing and nurse prescribing.

Many legal experts and authors express concerns as to whether Bolam is still relevant in the healthcare services of the 21st century since it effectively allows the medical profession to state the standard on which they will be judged. Simanowitz (1997) suggests that the validity of the Bolam test needs to be continuously 'attacked' by lawyers. He cites an Australian case, ***Rogers v Whitaker (1992)***, where a doctor was being sued following recanalisation after vasectomy that resulted in the patient's wife becoming pregnant. The defendant stated that he normally warned patients of the risk of recanalisation but omitted to do so, due to an oversight. Nevertheless, the doctor appealed to the Bolam principle, saying that a responsible body of doctors would not have informed patients of the risk. The court found in favour of the plaintiff, stating that 'The risk was so serious that the patient should have been warned'. Simanowitz concludes by stating that 'The Bolam principle provides a defence for those who lag behind the times'.

Stauch (1997) also supports the view that the courts appear to be taking a 'more critical' stance to doctors and cites the case of ***Bolitho v City and Hackney HA (1993)*** in which Lord Justice Farquharson suggested that

'Ultimately, the judge must decide whether a particular clinical practice, even one endorsed by a body of doctors, puts the patient unnecessarily at risk. Thus, while compliance with approved practice may make it unlikely that a doctor is guilty of negligence, it does not settle the matter'. Stauch refers to this development as the 'new Bolam'.

As stated, the Bolam test defines the standard as that of the reasonable person professing to have that same skill. However, what is not clear is whether the nurse taking on a role hitherto undertaken by doctors will be judged against the reasonable doctor or the reasonable nurse test. It may be that nursing and medical guidelines and standards would need to be referred to in attempts to determine the nature of the harm.

It appears that the law will focus on whether, in the performance of the role, the nurse achieved the level of competence demanded by the role. It is unlikely that the UKCC or the legal profession will accept as a defence that professional (nursing) accountability can be denied because the role was once a medical one. According to Bolam, it appears sufficient if the nurse exercises an ordinary level of care.

However, whilst this basic level of competency may satisfy the law, it is important for nurses to realise that in any scrutiny of professional standards, the UKCC may demand more than basic competence and may independently proceed against the nurse. Appropriate disciplinary action will be taken where the standards have, in the UKCC's view, not reached an acceptable professional level.

Elliott Pennels (1997) highlights that it is important to remember that the standard of care is related to 'the post and not to the individual ... that is, it is related to the skills that are needed for the job, not what skills the individual doing the job can offer'.

In the case of ***R v Bateman (1925)*** cited in Kennedy and Grubb (1989), Lord Hewart stated 'If a person holds himself out as possessing special skill and knowledge ... by or on behalf of a patient ... he owes a duty to the patient to use diligence, care, knowledge, skill and caution in administering the treatment'.

Whilst the legal principles discussed so far relate to doctors, the same principles would apply to nurses and nursing standards. This has particular significance for those who, like nurse prescribers, are undertaking roles traditionally performed by doctors.

POTENTIAL BREACHES OF DUTY OF CARE IN PRESCRIBING

It is essential that nurse prescribers, through continuous reflection on their prescribing role, identify areas where potential breaches of duty may occur. Potential breaches of duty could occur in:

- prescribing
- product liability
- consent
- communications.

Box 2.2 – Duty of care for the nurse prescriber involves personal accountability for:

- being adequately prepared for the role including attending an approved nurse-prescribing programme

- abiding by professional standards of care including the UKCC standards for the administration of medicines

- understanding the legal and professional basis (including the 'Bolam test') for determining the standard of care for safe prescribing and take appropriate actions to reduce that risk.

Prescribing

Areas of Prescribing which could potentially render the Nurse Prescriber vulnerable include:

- prescription writing
- preferential prescribing
- security of prescription pads.

Prescription writing

The writing of a prescription implies an acceptance by the nurse prescriber of personal accountability for knowledge of the patient's current and past medical history, current medications and knowledge of the side effects and contraindications for the products prescribed. 'The nurse who takes the original decision and writes the prescription is responsible in law for ensuring that the prescription is used in accordance with their instructions' (ENB, 1998: p. 2.2).

To ensure legal validity, the prescription must be legible, dated and signed. In addition, it must be appropriate, accurate, not contain any abbreviations and be based on products listed in the NPF. The prescriber is responsible for ensuring that all prescriptions are entered not only on the nurse or patient-held records but also in the General Practitioner GP-held records. If a decision is made not to prescribe, the reason should be recorded in the patient's records. The nurse prescriber also needs to be aware when it is more appropriate to refer a patient to the GP, rather than issue a prescription. If a nurse decides not to prescribe but recommends to the patient or client that they purchase the product over the counter (OTC), the nurse remains accountable for giving any relevant information concerning use and storage of the OTC product. The reason the nurse remains legally liable is because the advice is given within the therapeutic relationship existing between patient and nurse, which may influence the patient to preferentially purchase a particular product.

It is important that nurses should discuss prescribing role parameters with GPs to ensure that mutual agreement is reached on actions to be taken in the event of a disagreement over products prescribed. However, it is important to realise that 'In the event of a disagreement between professionals over treatment of a patient, the GP responsible for the care of the patient will, as at present, take the final decision' (DoH, 1989 cited in ENB, 1994).

Good record keeping in prescribing is not only essential to ensure safe continuity of care and identification of areas of risk for patients but also because, in the future, nurse prescribing could be one of the new developments assessed by the *National Institute of Clinical Effectiveness* (NICE). If the quality of record keeping is poor, it may prevent accurate assessment of the effectiveness of nurse prescribing in delivering an improved quality of service for patients. Poor record keeping may also hinder attempts to provide vital data should nurse prescribers in the future demand an extension of the NPF.

The quality of record keeping itself may be negatively affected by the repetitive data entries expected from nurse prescibers. Currently (and dependent on local procedures), many nurses are expected to separately enter details of the prescription in records held by the patient, the nurse, the parents and the GP. Nurse prescribers and managers should discuss these issues and devise systems which are 'practitioner and patient friendly' and which accord with legal and professional standards for record keeping.

Preferential prescribing

Nurse prescribers need to be aware of external influences on prescription choices as they may find themselves targeted in sales promotions by commercial firms.

Commercial representatives may attempt to persuade nurses to preferentially prescribe their products. If a product is preferentially prescribed, the nurse remains responsible for the appropriateness of the prescription which should include checking the claims made for the product in any sales promotion. This will involve the nurse reading all the sales promotional literature and, in particular, any data relating to research studies on which claims for the product are based.

As in all other areas, nurses need to be aware of the UKCC *Code of Professional Conduct*, which states that nurses' 'professional judgement is not influenced by commercial considerations'. In addition, nurses need to abide by their employers' policies and procedures on accepting and declaring any inducements to prescribe preferentially.

Preferential prescribing may involve the nurse prescriber in ethical issues which, if unresolved, may not only compromise professional practice, but render the practitioner legally vulnerable. For a fuller discussion of ethical issues see Chapter 3.

Security of prescription pads

Security of the individual prescription pad remains the responsibility of prescribers, who should also ensure that they do not lend the pad to others. Dependent on the circumstances, for example failure to ensure that the pad was stored securely, loss of the prescription pad could constitute a disciplinary offence under the employers' procedures.

Each prescription pad will have a 'new unique nurse identifier' (ENB, 1998) which in many areas is the nurse's UKCC personal identification number (PIN). The UKCC advises that nurses should retain their PIN numbers securely and that in the event of loss, the UKCC should be informed.

Many nurse prescribers are concerned that maintenance of PIN security is impossible if the PIN is written on a prescription which is then given to

> **Box 2.3 – The duty of care in relation to the prescription could potentially be breached in these areas**
>
> - Prescription writing
> - Preferential prescribing
> - Security of prescription pads

patients. In addition, they express concerns that loss of a prescription pad containing the PIN could expose them to personal and professional risk, as it may be possible for anyone who gains possession of it not only to access information held by the UKCC but to fraudulently use the PIN to gain employment. Medical prescriptions do not include the doctor's professional PIN.

Product liability

Nurse prescribers must be aware of their responsibilities for giving product information under the Consumer Protection Act 1987. This Act relates to the safety of products and creates strict liability for injuries caused by defective products. A defective product is defined by the Act as one which is '. . . not as safe as people are generally entitled to expect'. The concept of liability for products requires a complainant to demonstrate that a particular product is defective under the Act and that the product caused harm. Defective drugs come within the scope of the Act but 'a drug will only be "defective" where it can be shown that the risks associated with its use are so grave that they outweigh the potential benefits of treatment' (Korgaonakar and Tribe, 1995).

The Consumer Protection Act is drafted in such a way as to allow the complainant who is unable to identify the producer of the product to sue the person who supplied them with it. The definition of 'supplier' would include doctors, pharmacists and nurse prescribers.

The implications of this Act for nurse prescribers are that they are accountable for ensuring that information concerning the side effects and particular instructions regarding the product are given to the patient. Additionally, that information is given regarding the safe storage and disposal of prescribed products. It is good professional practice to record in the patient's notes that such information was given.

Consent

In law, any mentally competent adult has the right to consent to any touching of their person. Any non–consensual touching could result in a civil action for trespass to the person. Consent can be implied or expressed. An example of implied consent is where the patient's actions imply that they have given consent; for example, when a patient rolls up their sleeve on being informed that the nurse wishes to take their blood pressure. Expressed consent, given verbally or in writing, is an explicit consent to any invasive procedure or treatment or where there is a known risk element.

Nurse prescribers need to be aware of their professional and legal responsibility for giving sufficient information, on which a balanced judgement of whether to accept or refuse the treatment can be made. Expressed consent should be sought for any product which the nurse prescribes and intends to use invasively, e.g. urinary catheters. Where the patient is incapable of giving expressed consent, the nurse should advise relatives or carers of the reason for the prescription and treatment and record the information in the patient's records. Nurses should ensure that in the case of adults incapable of giving consent, decisions regarding any proposed treatment are made on the basis that it will be in the best interests of the patient. This decision may have to be justified at a later date.

Communicating with colleagues

The role of the nurse prescriber could potentially cause areas of disagreement or misunderstanding with other non-prescribing colleagues (including managers). Colleagues who do not fully understand the prescriber responsibilities may request prescriptions for their patients 'to save bothering the GP'. Such requests should be carefully considered. They involve prescribing for a patient who has not been assessed by the prescriber and they may have little or no knowledge of the patient.

It would be good practice for managers with staff who have successfully attended nurse prescriber courses to interview them on completion of the course to discuss these and other prescribing-related issues. Managers should be aware that vicarious liability may not be effective for nurse prescribers until they have been authorised in the role. Vicarious liability is defined in terms of the employer's liability for the negligence of employees acting in the course of their employment. Issues relating to aspects of the role should be fully discussed and role parameters clearly understood by

---

Box 2.4 – Areas in which breaches of the duty of care may occur

- **Prescribing**
The prescription should be valid and used in accordance with the nurse prescriber's instructions

- **Product liability**
Information about side effects and particular instructions regarding the product should be given to the patient

- **Consent**
Sufficient information should be given to the patient on which a decision to accept or refuse the treatment can be made

- **Communication**
Nurse prescribers should communicate effectively with colleagues on all aspects relating to individual prescriptions

---

both parties. In taking on the new role, the manager and prescriber should also carefully examine existing standards and protocols which may need to be revised and updated to reflect the new responsibility.

Nurses should also discuss the new role with other prescribing colleagues and agree actions to be taken in the event of any concerns with products prescribed by another nurse prescriber. In addition, the nurse prescriber should be aware of the Primary Care Group or Trust position on issues such as prescribing patterns and budgetary limits for prescribing.

CONCLUSION

It is clear that nurse prescribers have a duty of care to patients to ensure that:

- they are adequately prepared for the role

- they understand the legal and professional framework for the role

- they are competent in the performance of the role

- the standards of their prescribing care meet with professional and legal requirements.

As discussed earlier, the *Scope of Professional Practice* (UKCC, 1992a) expects that nurses should take appropriate steps to maintain role competence. This includes developing and maintaining their knowledge of 'pharmacology and the life sciences' (Courtenay and Butler, 1999).

Maintenance of competence and updating knowledge and skills can be done through a variety of mediums including:

- peer support
- auditing nurse prescribing
- reviewing prescribing patterns
- critical incident reviews
- clinical supervision
- keeping abreast with current prescribing literature.

Since the role of nurse prescribing is still relatively new, the new prescriber may experience a lack of peer support or clinical supervision. As this new role is traditionally a medical one, it may be appropriate for a doctor to act as clinical supervisor for the nurse prescriber, since they would be qualified to challenge the prescriber's decisions.

It is clear from the discussions in this chapter that nurse prescribers are professionally and legally accountable for every aspect of the prescribing process, including the knowledge base and practical skills. Nurses also need to be aware of social developments which may impact on prescribing practice; for example, their responsibility and accountability in prescribing for people such as those seeking political asylum who may not be registered with a GP. Equally, health visitors who run clinics for mothers and children who come from different geographical areas must be certain about their position in relation to prescribing.

As with any new development, nurses should be vigilant in reflecting on practice and attempt to identify the areas where patient safety may be compromised and, together with other prescribers and managers, devise appropriate procedures designed to reduce risk.

Box 2.5 – Some practice issues which nurse prescribers should consider

- How will performance in the role be assessed?

- Where and how will the patient's prescription be documented?

- How will the effectiveness of the prescription be evaluated?

- How will prescribing patterns be monitored?

- What actions should be taken in the event of needing to prescribe for patients
  - not registered with a GP?
  - not from the practitioner's catchment area?

- What is the procedure for adding a nurse-prescribed medicine to those already dispensed by a pharmacist in a sealed monitored dosage system?

Cases

Bolam vs Friern Barnet Hospital Management Committee (1957) 2 ALL ER 118
Medical Bolitho vs City and Hackney HA (1993)
Blyth vs Birmingham Water Works (1856) 11 Exch
Donoghue v Stevenson (1932) AC 562
Nettleship v Weston (1971) ALL ER 581; (1971) 3 WLR 370
R v Bateman (1925) LJKB 791, CCA
Rogers v Whitaker (1992) 3 Med LR 331

Statutes

Consumer Protection Act 1987
Medicines Act 1968
Medicinal Products: Prescription by Nurses etc Act 1992
Pharmaceutical Services Regulations 1994

References

Courtenay, M. & Butler, M. (1999). *Nurse Prescribing: Principles and Practice*. London: Greenwich Medical Media.

Department of Health (1999). *Review of Prescribing, Supply and Administration of Medicines* (Crown Report). London: Department of Health.

Dimond, B. (1995). *Legal Aspects of Nursing*. London: Prentice Hall. P 28

Elliott Pennels, C. (1997). Professional negligence. *Professional Nurse* 13(1): Pages 50–53

English National Board for Nursing, Midwifery and Health Visiting (1998*). Nurse Prescribing Open Learning Pack*. Milton Keynes: Learning Materials Design. P 59

Kennedy, I. & Grubb, A. (1989). *Medical Law Text and Materials*. London: Butterworths. P 396

Korgaonaker, G. & Tribe, D. (1995). *Law for Nurses*. Cavendish Publishing. London. P 147

Rieu, S. Error and Trial, The Extended Role Dilemma. *British Journal of Nursing*, 1994 3(4) P 168–174

Simanowitz, A. Editorial AV-MA Medical and Legal Journal

Stauch, M. (1997). The legal concept of medical negligence, *British Journal of Nursing* 6(22): 1325.

Tingle, J. (1990). Accountability and the law: how it affects the nurse. *Senior Nurse* 10(2): 8–9.

Tingle, J. & Cribb, A. (1995). *Nursing Law and Ethics*. Oxford: Blackwell Science. P 143

United Kingdom Central Council for Nursing, Midwifery and Health Visiting (1992a). *The Scope of Professional Pratice*. London: UKCC.

United Kingdom Central Council for Nursing, Midwifery and Health Visiting (1992b). *The Code of Professional Conduct*. London: UKCC.

3

ETHICAL ISSUES IN NURSE PRESCRIBING

INTRODUCTION

We use the word 'issue' in a variety of ways. To draw attention to the significance of some matter, we may 'raise it as an issue', to deny its significance we may say 'For me it simply isn't an issue'. If it turns out not to be significant, it 'ceases to be an issue'. So identifying something 'as an issue' is not a neutral, merely objective, matter: evaluation is involved and, implicitly at least, values which confer significance.

In this sense, nurse prescribing has highlighted a range of issues and to single some of these out as 'ethical' is to imply that the values involved are those that shape good professional practice, whether these are explicit in codes and guidelines or implicit as underlying moral principles.

Given a basis of shared professional values, it is not surprising that there is a broad consensus as to what the ethical issues are. Neither are these issues radically new; rather, it is a case of familiar themes arising in a new context – themes such as accountability, confidentiality and relations with clients.

Shared professional values enter into the equation in at least two other ways. Many of the issues arise out of a tension between values: for example, between concern for a patient's well-being and a duty to respect their autonomy. Values delimit the scope of permissible debate; unsafe practice, for example, is not an option.

In describing the ethical issues involved in nurse prescribing, then, this chapter will highlight the values involved. However, since anything that is an issue is, potentially at least, a matter for debate, my intention is also to get into the debate.

RULES, GUIDELINES AND PRINCIPLES

The practice of nurse prescribing takes place within the context of rules. There are legal rules, for example the law prohibiting the use of items in the boot of your car prescribed for other patients, but no longer wanted by them; professional rules, such as that requiring that a prescription should be written only on the basis of the prescriber's own assessment of the patient; and protocols, specifying procedure in relation to the issuing of prescriptions. Anecdotal evidence indicates that in some areas the use of protocols is not now favoured. Whether a rejection of protocols as a means of structuring nurse prescribing becomes widespread remains to be seen.

Whereas guidelines allow scope for discretion and the exercise of judgement, rules, it might seem, give no such scope. Nevertheless, where practice is constrained by rules, the practitioner may wish to query their status and ask whether they do indeed allow for no exceptions; in other words, whether they are absolute. This query may arise out of the demands of practice and it is clearly a question with implications for practice. One way of assessing the status of these rules is to determine their justification and an answer to this brings principles into the picture.

This is illustrated by a scenario imagined by Cooper (1993). A man is out driving with his children. He stops at a red traffic light and his young daughter wants to know why he's stopped. He explains he had to; the rule is, cars have to stop when the lights are at red. His teenage son (a budding philosopher!) asks 'But why do we have to have rules anyway?'. The father's explanation appeals to fairness ('Since people who drive have a right to share the highway, it is only fair that they should get their turn to cross this busy intersection'), and to non-maleficence ('If the rules let everyone cross whenever they want to, they may crash into each other').

Cooper thus uses the scenario to illustrate a view that rules are justified, if at all, by reference to underlying principles and he offers the diagram in **Figure 3.1**.

In querying the rules that constrain nurse prescribing, then, practitioners may find that they are justified by reference to underlying principles. For example, in respect of the rules mentioned earlier, the legal rule against using prescribed treatments kept in your boot may be justified by reference to the principle of harm (non-maleficence) because treatments that are out of date or that are not used for the named patient or that may not now correspond to their label may be unsafe; and the professional rule that

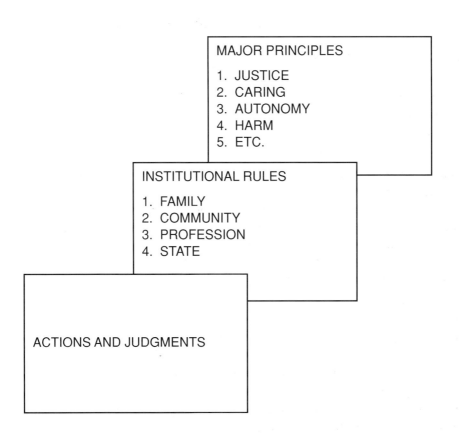

Figure 3.1 – The link between actions and judgments, institutional rules and principles.

prescribing must be on the basis of assessment by the prescribing nurse may be justified by reference to the principle of professional accountability (see Chapter 2).

So much for the question of justification. This suggests an answer to the other question, i.e. whether the rules are absolute, applying in all possible circumstances. The answer is this: exceptions may be justifiable when, in the circumstances, the principle underpinning the rule is judged to favour an exception to that rule or when another principle, perceived as more important in the circumstances than the principle underpinning the rule, is judged to favour an exception.

Cooper's scenario can be developed to illustrate this. In a crisis, where a person's life depends on speed, an ambulance will go through the lights at red. This exception to the rule can be justified either by the claim that, in this case, the principle of harm underpinning the rule (which highlights the danger if the rule is broken) favours breaking the rule (because of the danger to the patient in the ambulance if the rule is not broken) or by the claim that, in this case, the principle of fairness that also underpins the rule (everyone waiting their turn) is less important than the principle of non-maleficence (the danger of harm to the patient).

Two nurse-prescribing scenarios can illustrate this and bring us back to the realities of practice.

Scenario 1

A district nurse who is a qualified nurse prescriber is asked by a colleague with a particularly heavy caseload to visit a client who needs a leg ulcer dressing changed. The nurse visits the client and on assessing the wound, decides that the current dressing is inappropriate. When she tells the client that a different dressing would be better, the client is anxious to continue with the dressing already used. However, the nurse discovers that there are no dressings left.

Discussion of this scenario with students preparing for the nurse-prescribing examination revealed that a serious option for many would be to fetch a dressing from their car. This was justified by reference to the client's immediate need (she couldn't be left with an open wound) and the judgement that the particular dressing available is safe. In this case, therefore, it may be claimed that the principle of harm underpinning the legal rule favours an exception to the rule.

Scenario 2

A district nurse prescriber is a team manager. She has prescribed a dressing for a client on the basis of her own assessment and appointed a member of her team to carry out the care. Having seen the client, her colleague – who is an expert in wound care – suggests that the prescription should be changed to a similar product. The manager writes out a different prescription, on her colleague's advice.

Strictly applied, the rules require that the team manager make another visit. It may be, however, that in this situation it would be justifiable for her to prescribe on her colleague's advice. The practicalities may be that she is massively busy, both as a manager and as a nurse, with a heavy caseload, and she is aware of her colleague's expertise. As we have seen, the rule which precludes her action is justified by reference to professional accountability: however, in this case, it might be argued that, in making an exception to the rule, she has acted both accountably and responsibly.

Before moving on, perhaps it should be said, that in raising the possibility that rules might have exceptions and in identifying situations where this may be the case, I do not mean to downplay the importance of rules. Rules have an essential role in structuring practice and I am aware, in particular, of the importance currently attached to the rule requiring that a nurse who prescribes should herself make the assessment (a student who called this in question would, in my experience, fail the qualifying examination). Rather, I want to acknowledge that in the realities of concrete situations, in which other values may play a part, the practitioner may have to make a judgement. In this acknowledgement there is an implicit claim – that ethical practice is not synonymous with rule following.

ISSUES OF CONFIDENTIALITY

Situations that may arise in relation to confidentiality in nurse prescribing illustrate both a clear application of a rule to practice (here, the rule that information relating to clients should be kept confidential) and also scope for debate as to how the rule applies. This again can be highlighted in two scenarios.

Scenario 1

On the caseload of a health visitor who is a qualified nurse prescriber are two clients, Anne Marie and her close friend, Sara. Anne Marie is a single parent with two small children, Jamie aged two years and eight-month-old Becky. Anne Marie has recently returned to part-time work and is able to do this because her mother looks after the children. However, she is feeling exhausted because Becky is teething, crying at night and keeping her awake. Sara has told her friend that the health visitor prescribed Calpol for her son and, prompted by this, Anne Marie asks for a prescription of Calpol for Becky. When the health visitor refuses, Anne Marie gets angry, pointing out that she had prescribed Calpol for Sara's son.

In the course of a potentially heated exchange, the health visitor is under pressure to comment, by way of explanation, on her dealings with Sara. The temptation to comment may be the stronger because she knows that Anne Marie and Sara don't have secrets from each other and that Anne Marie may well be privy to what she had said to Sara.

Nevertheless, discussion with nurses indicates a professional consensus that the health visitor would be right not to comment, she would be right to adhere strictly to the rule of confidentiality. By adhering to the rule, she upholds an important moral principle – from which the rule in part derives its force, i.e. respect for privacy.

(I am grateful to Caroline Packham for this scenario.)

Scenario 2

A district nurse prescriber doing weekend cover prescribes for patients from six surgeries. She has to enter records of the prescriptions at each surgery within 48 hours. The surgeries are situated over a wide area. The time involved in visits to all six would therefore be considerable. As she is a community nurse with a heavy caseload, she faxes a copy of the prescription, thus saving precious time.

The rights and wrongs of this scenario can be debated in terms of the tension between a duty to manage time effectively, based on the nurse's accountability to the patients on her own caseload, and a duty to keep patients' records confidential. However, to set up the debate in these terms presupposes that faxing records does constitute, or at least risk, a breach of confidentiality but this is itself open to debate. For the presupposition ignores practical matters, like where the fax machine is placed and who has access to it; it also depends on a particular understanding of the scope of confidentiality, in assuming that should receptionists have access to faxed information, there would be a breach. In this regard, it could be argued that, although general practice receptionists are not under the same professional discipline as nurses, they are contractually under a duty of confidentiality, are in an important sense part of the team and that therefore should they gain access to private information, there is not necessarily a breach.

Even if it is judged that faxing does constitute or risk a breach of confidentiality, the question of what, in this case, is justifiable ethically remains open. If the dilemma is posed in general terms, i.e. without reference to the particularities of a given situation, a clear answer is not readily available, for how in general does one 'weigh' a concern about confidentiality against a concern about effective and accountable use of time? In practice, however, dilemmas don't arise 'in general terms' but in particular situations and it may be that the concrete details of each of these indicate a way through. For example, in a given situation, what at the start of *this* week are the demands on the nurse? Are there patients on *this* Monday morning who are likely to have particularly urgent needs, which will mean that her time is at a premium? Or not? What are the details of the prescriptions she has written over this weekend? Do any convey rather sensitive information? Or not? Are other surgeries known to be somewhat lax or is there careful practice in relation to keeping information confidential?

These reflections highlight what I take to be the familiar fact that, in practice, dilemmas have to be worked through by the exercise of judgement and attention to the particularities of each situation; and as practitioners know, they can be and are worked through.

MONEY MATTERS

Other issues requiring the 'exercise of judgement and attention to the particularities of each situation' are raised by the cost of prescriptions. These are highlighted in the following scenarios.

Scenario 1

A nurse, working with a client who was not exempt from prescription charges, advised her client to buy an emollient cream over the counter. She did not prescribe in this case, because she believed her client was not well off and knew that the prescription would cost more.

Scenario 2

A nurse prescribed paracetamol for a client although she felt that ibuprofen, not available on prescription, would have been more appropriate. She did this believing that the client was poor and could ill afford to buy ibuprofen.

Scenario 3

A health visitor did not prescribe paracetamol for a baby. Although she felt it was the appropriate treatment for the baby's condition, she advised the mother to buy paracetamol over the counter, believing the mother was well able to afford it.

In all three scenarios, the nurse makes an assessment of what the client can afford. On the basis of her assessment, in the first she acts to protect the client, in the second she prescribes treatment that is less than ideal and in the third she acts to protect the budget.

One issue arising is whether such assessment should be part of a nurse prescriber's brief. This again is something that has come up for discussion amongst nurses preparing for the nurse-prescribing qualification. Two views are typically put forward: one that this is part of an holistic approach and therefore right and proper, the other that it is easy to get it wrong (clients, it is claimed, may appear to be well off and yet be strapped for cash or appear to be hard up and yet in fact be well off) and therefore that it is dangerous territory. These views, though, are not mutually exclusive: one could accept that assessing what a client can afford is justifiable in principle and also acknowledge that in practice it may be difficult to get it right. The element of risk (the risk of getting it wrong) is no doubt minimised where the client is well known to the nurse.

Another issue arising from the scenarios is whether awareness of the cost of prescriptions should shape a nurse's treatment of patients in any way and if it should, in what way.

As regards the first question (whether awareness of the cost of prescriptions should shape a nurse's treatment of patients in any way), the fact that prescribing takes place in a context of limited resources means that, in principle, awareness of cost should be a factor; however, as regards the second (how this may justifiably shape her treatment of individual patients) there is scope for debate. Would denying a client's right to free prescriptions (as in the third scenario) be acceptable? Intuitively, this feels hard to justify. Would providing a treatment that is less than ideal be acceptable? Intuitively, this also feels hard to justify and the intuition, on inspection, arises out of a sense of the values implicit in a nurse's relationship with her client. In some circumstances, the dilemma may be dissolved by the fact that treatment that is initially more costly may over time be less expensive than a cheaper one, as it is effective more quickly.

What is clear is that, given limited resources, prescribing that wastes resources is not justifiable. An example of waste would be if a district nurse were to prescribe a four layer dressing for a leg ulcer knowing the patient wouldn't stay with it. Another example would be if a prescription for head lice were written for a child whose parents, not exempt from prescription charges, could not afford to buy treatment for themselves because, in such a case, to treat one member of the family only would be futile.

In this section, reference has been made in passing to the values implicit in a nurse's relationship with her client. This theme is highlighted also in the section below.

ISSUES OF CARE AND COMPLIANCE

Nurses have a duty to care for their patients (see Chapter 2) and they care about their patients. They also in an important sense know best; that is, they know what is the best and most appropriate treatment for specific conditions. So there is an issue when their knowledge is, in effect, discounted and the patient refuses or is reluctant to go along with their advice. This is illustrated in the following scenarios.

Scenario 1

A female patient refused to accept the nurse's advice that she should wear compression hosiery. She said 'It would threaten my lifestyle'.

Scenario 2

A male patient had been coming to the surgery regularly for months for treatment for his leg ulcer. The ulcer had now healed. The nurse advised him that if he didn't wear compression hosiery, the ulcer would return. The man (who was known to the surgery as an 'awkward customer') refused, saying she didn't know his body as he did. He continued to attend the surgery every week, at the same time, for the nurse to look at his leg.

Scenario 3

An elderly female patient had been having treatment for her leg ulcer for some time. The treatment had not been very successful. A nurse newly assigned to her care proposed a change of treatment, recommending that a four layer bandage be used instead. The patient was reluctant to change.

All three scenarios raise issues of care and compliance. I use the first to illustrate the fact that non-compliance may set a limit on a nurse's responsibility: the nurse commented 'There was nothing I could do'. The second is a situation where a judgement has to be made as to how to continue to work with a non-compliant patient and raises the question of the point at which a nurse has discharged her responsibility. In this particular case, the nurse judged that the man was lonely, that he liked the fixed routine to which he'd become accustomed of attending the surgery every week and that he valued (needed?) the attention he found there. Medically, this was no longer needed; holistically, maybe it was. The third is a situation where the nurse has to judge whether to try to persuade the patient to accept her advice and if so, how to do this. Needless to say, respect for the patient means she can't simply overrule her reluctance and impose the new treatment; in any case, if she did this it would possibly be counterproductive as the patient might remove the dressing when she'd gone. The same outcome might ensue if, as a result of talk and gentle persuasion there was only half-hearted assent. Whether in such circumstances the patient has given genuine consent may be difficult to judge. Much depends on how well nurse and patient know each other and how much trust there is in the relationship.

If this particular discussion seems inconclusive, this is perhaps inevitable, since there is a limit to what can usefully be said in general about such difficult practical matters. As was claimed earlier, dilemmas of practice can only be worked through 'by judgement and by attention to the particularities of each situation'.

ISSUES OF RESPONSIBILITY

There is a sense in which all the issues so far discussed are issues of responsibility, all are areas of ethical concern in which practitioners have to exercise responsibility. However, what I want to highlight now is a particular issue relating to the scope of responsibility for outcomes.

The Nurse Prescribing Open Learning Pack (ENB, 1998) notes that 'Nurses are responsible not only for the care that they give but also for the care given by others as a result of a nursing decision'. The pack goes on to state that:

'This is very relevant to nurse prescribing as, in the community, substances or dressings prescribed by the nurse will often be applied or administered by someone else, such as the patient, a carer, or a health care assistant. The nurse who takes the original decision and writes the prescription is responsible in law for ensuring that the prescription is used in accordance with their instructions.' (p. 2.2)

The ethical question here is, if things go wrong, in what circumstances would it be morally justifiable to say the prescribing nurse is responsible? To pursue this question, one has to be precise as to what might be meant by saying the nurse is responsible and to distinguish between different uses of the word 'responsible'.

Role responsibility

To say that a nurse is responsible for something may imply that it is one of the obligations or duties assigned to her – that thing is one of her responsibilities. This is presumably what is meant when it is said (as above) that 'nurses are responsible ... for the care given by others', and that they are 'responsible in law for ensuring that the prescription is used in accordance with their instructions'.

Causal responsibility

To say that a nurse is responsible for something may imply that some outcome is a result of what she did or did not do. In other words, what she did or did not do caused it. (Causal responsibility may be shared: there may be, and perhaps typically are, a variety of causal factors behind any given outcome.)

Moral responsibility

To say that a nurse is (causally) responsible for something does not necessarily suggest that it was her fault, i.e. that she is morally responsible. In other words, the outcome may be a result of what she did or did not do but it may be unjustified to blame her, to 'hold her responsible'.

When a nurse writes a prescription and things go wrong, there is a straightforward sense in which she must be causally responsible – at least in part – for the outcome: if she hadn't written the prescription, things would have been different! But she may not be morally responsible, i.e. she may not be to blame. There are at least two mitigating conditions: (i) unavoidable ignorance and (ii) incapacity.

(i) Unavoidable ignorance

Perhaps there were factors she couldn't have known about when writing the prescription. For example, a district nurse doing cover duty may not have access to a patient's medical notes and, when asked, the patient, by oversight, may not tell her what other medication he or she is taking.

(ii) Incapacity

Perhaps situations arise where there is nothing she can do. For example, a young mother who has been prescribed aspirin absent-mindedly leaves the bottle open on the kitchen table. Her three-year-old child sees the bottle and swallows some, wanting to copy mummy.

So, to answer the ethical question posed above ('In what circumstances would it be morally justifiable to say the prescribing nurse is responsible?'), the nurse is only justifiably held to be (morally) responsible if she could have known of the factors that, in the event, led to a bad outcome or if she could have acted to prevent it and failed to do so.

These examples show that there is a sense in which a nurse prescriber cannot 'ensure' that a prescription is used in accordance with her instructions. This is not to deny that there is much she can do to make it highly probable that things will go well and good practice in this respect is, arguably, all that can be expected of the practitioner.

To highlight 'good practice' is to bring into view careful, diligent, practice in which, for example, the prescribing nurse checks out what other medication a patient may be taking and makes every effort to ensure that the patient understands what the treatment involves. (Needless to say, a careful, diligent practitioner would have explained to the mother in the above scenario that aspirin can be dangerous, especially to young children.)

To highlight good practice is also to bring into view the nurse as an accountable practitioner, accountable to her patient and to her profession.

CONCLUSION

This discussion has touched on, and to some extent debated, a number of ethical issues in nurse prescribing. There are of course others which, for reasons of space, have not been mentioned. An emergent theme has been the need for judgement and it may be useful, by way of conclusion, to draw on the discussion to highlight factors which may inform the practitioner's judgement in a given situation.

Though it was claimed that ethical practice is not morally equivalent to rule following, the importance of rules in constraining nurse prescribing was affirmed. Reference was also made to the significance of outcomes and of the values implicit in a good relationship with patients and clients. That care – caring for and caring about patients and clients – is integral to nursing was noted. Nurses may find that in working through dilemmas involved in nurse prescribing 'by the exercise of judgement and attention to the particularities of each situation', any or all of these factors may come into play.

Acknowledgements

I am indebted to students and to my colleagues Deborah Stevens and Kathleen Hutchinson at the University of Reading and to Lois Goding at Buckinghamshire Chilterns University College, for sharing their practical experience and their understanding of nurse prescribing with me, and to Lois Goding for her comments on a first draft of this chapter.

References

Cooper, D. (1993). *Value Pluralism and Ethical Choice*. New York: St Martin's Press.

English National Board for Nursing, Midwifery and Health Visiting (1998). *Nurse Prescribing Open Learning Pack*. Milton Keynes: Learning Materials Design.

4

CLINICAL DIAGNOSIS AND MANAGEMENT FOR THE NURSE PRESCRIBER

INTRODUCTION

This chapter is written by an inner-city GP who teaches part of a basic nurse prescriber course. The subject matter reflects the content of the course modified by feedback from participants. When specific treatment regimens are recommended, these are based on the best available clinical trial evidence. The chapter will concentrate on:

- itchy/scaly rashes (including atopic dermatitis and fungal infections)
- scabies
- head lice
- nappy rash
- constipation
- threadworms
- boils and carbuncles

- oral thrush

- ear wax.

Like most GPs, I welcome the introduction of nurse prescribing and the plans for its extension. GPs recognise that nurses are often best placed to diagnose and manage a range of clinical conditions and that prescribing can form part of this management.

COMMUNICATION

As nurse prescribing develops, it will become increasingly important that good channels of communication (both formal and informal) are set up between nurse prescribers and the practice teams with which they work as well as with local primary care groups (PCG/Ts) or primary care trusts (PCTs). Nurse prescribers should seek, and are entitled to expect, feedback and support relating to their prescribing from nursing, medical and pharmacy colleagues.

Communication needs to be maintained with community pharmacists (see Chapter 5), who may wish to contact the prescriber in the event of a query. It is important to make sure that the telephone number recorded in the box at the bottom of the prescription forms is appropriate.

Much useful information can be exchanged via the patient's clinical record. Duplication of recording is time consuming and likely to be prone to errors. I hope that, as trust and confidence grow, community nurses, health visitors and the general practice team will develop a single, common, primary care record system.

PRESCRIBING BUDGETS

Most products in the Nurse Prescribers' Formulary (NPF) are relatively inexpensive and it is anticipated that, in the next year or two, nurse prescriptions will account for only 1% of the budget for community prescribing. However, PCG/Ts and PCTs now have to work to fixed annual prescribing budgets and they are likely to scrutinise the Prescription Analysis and Cost (PACT) data for nurse prescribers (see Chapter 5). They will be keen to ensure that all prescribing is cost effective. Information on cost effectiveness is currently available from a number of periodicals and databases (e.g. Drugs and Therapeutics Bulletin, MeReC Bulletin, Clinical Evidence, Cochrane Database, Best Evidence, Bandolier, Evidence Based Nursing). In future, it is planned that the National Institute of Clinical Excellence (NICE) will issue guidelines and cost effectiveness data will be available via NHSNet. In an attempt to rationalise prescribing at a local level, PCG/Ts and primary care teams are being encouraged to develop their own local formularies and guidelines (see Chapter 5). Nurse prescribers need to be aware of these documents. The local PCG/T prescribing adviser (see Chapter 5) would be a good person to contact if seeking assistance.

The NHS medicines' budget is not intended to stock 'the family medicine chest' or for toiletry or cosmetic purposes. The prescribing rules require that prescriptions should be written to treat a specific medical condition in a particular patient. Nevertheless, the boundary between toiletries, cosmetics and medicines is sometimes unclear. Emollients are useful for dry skin but are they always 'medicines'? In an effort to limit prescribing, some PCG/Ts may introduce prescribing guidelines for such preparations: others will leave the decision to the individual prescriber.

CLINICAL EXAMINATION AND DIAGNOSIS

Accurate diagnosis is clearly a precursor to appropriate clinical management. Nurse prescribers may wish to enhance their examination skills in some clinical areas such as skin or ears; appropriate training should form part of continuing professional development. Primary care teams and PCG/Ts should consider these training needs within their overall educational plans. Examination skills training can be obtained on formal courses, but it may also be available informally locally.

REFERRAL

The decision to refer a patient to a nurse colleague, GP or hospital will be influenced by clinical, social and professional factors. It is impossible to give hard and fast rules on when to refer, but some reasons are listed below.

- Doubt about diagnosis
- Failure to resolve or an atypical response to treatment

- Adverse reactions to treatment

- The possibility of a complicating condition.

The cardinal rule of therapeutics is: *Non nocere* (do no harm). All the preparations in the NPF are safe if used appropriately.

RASHES

Diagnosis

Diffuse, itchy or scaly rashes are common, particularly in children and the elderly. Diagnosis is often difficult and imprecise and sometimes a pragmatic approach to therapy is appropriate. Many acute viral illnesses produce rashes that are red and may take the form of flat blotches *(macules)* or small raised lumps *(papules)*. Infections should be suspected in patients who have a fever and/or other systemic symptoms.

Common differential diagnoses for more chronic or subacute rashes include atopic dermatitis (**Figure 4.1**) and other eczemas, ringworm (**Figure 4.2**) and psoriasis (**Figure 4.3**). Rarer rashes that involve one or two patches include mycosis fungoides (a cutaneous lymphoma), solar keratoses (a premalignant condition related to sun damage) and Bowen's disease (a neoplastic condition associated with sun exposure). Nurse prescribers do not need to be able to diagnose these uncommon, more serious conditions but they do need to consider the possibility of their existence and refer rashes that exhibit atypical behaviour or appearance.

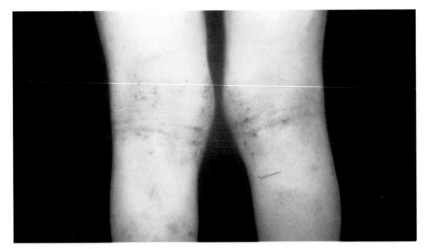

Figure 4.1 – Chronic excoriated atopic dermatitis.

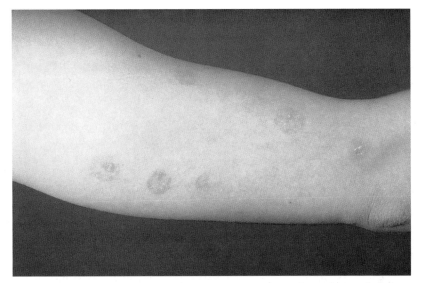

Figure 4.2 – Ringworm (*Tinea*) showing an active, red scaly edge and central clearing

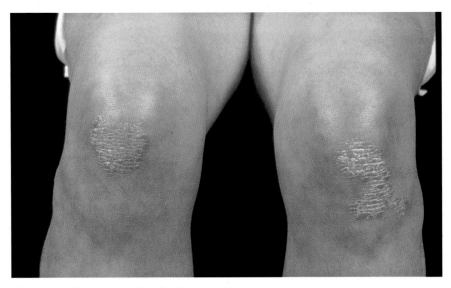

Figure 4.3 – Psoriasis – red, scaly plaques on knees.

History of the rash

Important features in the history are as follows.

- <u>Does the rash itch?</u> Most scaly rashes exhibit some itch but intense itchiness (*pruritus*) is more characteristic of atopic dermatitis, allergic dermatitis and scabies than the other conditions

- <u>What is the time course of the condition?</u> Atopic dermatitis and seborrhoeic eczema are chronic conditions whereas ringworm and allergic eczema present in just a few days

- <u>Family history</u> Atopic dermatitis runs in families

- <u>Is there any history of asthma?</u> Many atopic dermatitis sufferers also have asthma

- <u>Are any other members of the household affected?</u> Ringworm frequently affects more than one member of the family or school friends

- <u>Have any treatments already been tried?</u> Patients, or their parents, may have already consulted a pharmacist or used an 'over-the-counter' (OTC) topical preparation such as an emollient, steroid or antifungal cream. If steroids are inadvertently applied to fungal infections, the rash can become more widespread and atypical in appearance (*tinea incognito*).

Allergic contact dermatitis can be induced by many perfumes, preservatives and other materials in topical applications. Such allergens include lanolin, an ingredient of many emollients such as E45 cream and Keri lotion, and acharis (peanut) oil which is contained in Oilatum cream, Hydromol cream and oily calamine lotion. Allergy is usually acquired by repeated exposure to the allergen, so contact dermatitis can arise in patients who have been using a topical application for many years.

The itch of scabies can persist for a couple of weeks after successful eradication of the live mite. This can sometimes lead to repeated application of a scabicide with the subsequent development of contact dermatitis.

Examination

When examining a rash, the following features are important.

- <u>Distribution of the rash on the body</u>. Ringworm typically affects the limbs and flexures, whereas scabies is most commonly seen on the limbs and genitalia. The distribution of atopic dermatitis varies with age (see below)

- <u>The size and shape of discrete lesions</u>. The lesions of ringworm are typically annular

- <u>Is the rash flat or raised?</u> Atopic dermatitis is generally flat, except when the skin has been thickened by chronic scratching (lichenification), whereas psoriasis presents with raised plaques

- <u>The appearance of the surface of the rash (is it scaly, smooth or shiny?)</u>. Ringworm, psoriasis and seborrhoeic dermatitis are generally scaly whereas atopic dermatitis may be relatively smooth

- <u>The edge of lesion (is it clearly defined or graded?)</u> Patches of ringworm and psoriasis exhibit a well-demarcated edge, whereas in atopic dermatitis, the rash tends to blend into the surrounding normal skin (graded edge).

What is eczema?

The term 'eczema' is a generic term used to describe inflammatory rashes that involve oedema of the epidermis (Marks, 1993). Common eczemas relevant to nurse prescribers include:

- atopic dermatitis (unknown cause, probably immunological mediation)

- seborrhoeic dermatitis (probably has a microbial cause with overgrowth of skin flora)

- venous eczema (multiple causes but associated with gravitational stasis in the lower limbs and commonly progressing to venous ulceration)

- allergic contact dermatitis (delayed hypersensitivity reaction, can occur with topical medicaments, cosmetics, perfumes and lanolin).

Table 4.1 – *Clinical features of some common rashes that may be treated by nurse prescribers*

	Atopic dermatitis	Seborrhoeic dermatitis	Ringworm	Psoriasis	Scabies
Distribution	Depends on age, see Box 4.1	Scalp, flexures, face around nose, eyebrows, behind ears and nappy area	Extremities, trunk and flexures	Extensor surfaces, buttocks and flexures	Hands/feet genitalia, flexures and breasts (women)
Age ranges	Mainly babies and children	Commonest in babies and the elderly	Children of school age	Commonest in adults	Mainly teenagers and children, particularly in residential institutions
Itchy	Very	Slight	Slight	Minimal	Intensely
Scaly	Sometimes	Yes	Yes	Very	Rarely
Shape of lesion	Patches, usually flat	Flat patches	Annular patches, usually flat but may be raised in animal ringworm	Raised plaques	Papules or linear burrows, often with evidence of excoriation
Edge of lesion	Graded	Graded	Clearly defined	Clearly defined	
Other distinguishing features	Thickened (lichenified) areas of skin if chronic	May indicate immunosuppression (e.g. HIV)	Appearance may be untypical if patient has been treated with topical steroids	NA	NA
Associations	Asthma	NA	Other close contacts may have same	Smoking Stress	Other close contacts may have same

Atopic dermatitis (**Atopic eczema**)

Atopic dermatitis **(Figure 4.1)** is very common (10–15% of the population) and primarily occurs in infants and children (Rudikoff and Lebwohl, 1998). The distribution of the rash is dependent on the age of the patient and is shown in Box 4.1.

Emollients and bath oils are useful initial treatments for atopic dermatitis but in all but the mildest cases, topical steroids are also needed.

Box 4.1 – Distribution of atopic dermatitis

Infants (up to age 2)	Affects the cheeks and extensor parts of extremities; it sometimes shows weepy patches (exudation).
Childhood (age 2–12)	Raised lumps (*papulation*) rather than exudation and occurs in the flexures (behind the knees and at the elbows) and around the wrists, ankles and neck. Thickened, raised areas (*lichenification*) may occur at the sites of scratching. In black children, changes in the degree of pigmentation may be apparent.
Adults (from puberty onwards)	Characterised by lichenification of the flexures, wrists, ankles, feet, fingers and toes. The forehead may also be involved.

Seborrhoeic dermatitis

Seborrhoeic dermatitis is often difficult to distinguish from atopic dermatitis and fungal infections. It tends to be characterised by an itchy and scaly rash in the flexures around the hair line, nose and ears and over the eyebrows. It tends to occur in the young and the elderly. In infants, it can affect the nappy area. Seborrhoeic dermatitis is associated with an overgrowth of skin flora, particularly yeasts. A severe form is also associated with human immunodeficiency virus (HIV) infection. The condition is generally treated by combining an anti-yeast preparation (e.g. a topical imidazole) with a steroid cream (not currently in the NPF).

Fungal infections

The classic expanding annular appearance of skin fungal infections (ringworm), with an active inflamed edge and a pale centre, is well known **(Figure 4.2)**. However, fungi may also form a regular patch, not unlike eczema.

Examination of the edge of the lesion with a hand lens may aid diagnosis. Eczematous rashes tend to have a graded edge, whilst in fungal infections, the edge is well demarcated. Human forms of ringworm are generally quite flat, whilst ringworm caught from animals (usually household pets) is often raised and inflamed.

Fungal infections can be diagnosed by taking skin scrapings from the edge of the lesion and sending these to the pathology laboratory for mycological examination. Microscopic examination of the specimen may show fungal roots (*hyphae*) and takes just a few minutes to perform but culture of a fungus requires several weeks' incubation. Treatment with an imidazole cream or ointment would normally be started whilst awaiting the mycology result.

Pragmatic management of itchy/scaly rashes

It is important to consider and exclude, at an early stage, the possibility of skin cancer. Features that should make the clinician consider or suspect malignancy are:

- failure to respond to treatment
- bleeding or ulceration
- progressive enlargement
- a raised edge
- changes in pigmentation, particularly darkening
- blood vessels visible on the surface of the lesion.

The diagnosis of itchy/scaly rashes may be difficult at an early stage. Where fungal infections are suspected, mycological testing is recommended. In some cases, conservative treatment using an emollient or topical antifungal may be appropriate before diagnosis is certain. Timely review to assess the progress of treatment is recommended when treating rashes. Failure to respond to treatment would normally be an indication for referral to a GP.

For dry rashes, emollient ointments are better than creams for rehydrating skin. Unfortunately, many patients find ointments greasy and unpleasant and consequently fail to use them regularly. In such cases, it may be better to use a cream that is less efficacious but more acceptable; this is more likely to be applied regularly.

The quantities of emollient needed for various body parts are listed in the British National Formulary (BNF) (section 13.1.2) (Mehta, 2000). If the skin remains dry after a few days, emollient use should be monitored; the quantity and frequency of application are often inadequate. A useful additional treatment to emollient creams is bath oil but this is potentially hazardous for patients who might be prone to slip and slide when bathing.

Steroid creams (not currently part of the nurse formulary but available OTC) are indicated for all but the mildest forms of eczema. However, if topical steroids are inadvertently applied to fungal infections, the rash can become more widespread and atypical in appearance (*tinea incognito*).

Scalp and nail ringworm

Hair loss and scaly or boggy patches (kerions) on the head may be indicative of fungal infections of the scalp; deformation or discolouration of the nails is typical of onychomycosis (fungal nail infection).

In both these conditions, fungus is present deep within the affected tissue and topical treatment is generally ineffective. Systemic antifungal treatment (not currently in the NPF) is indicated after the diagnosis has been confirmed by mycological examination of samples (hair or nail clippings).

Spores shed from the head can cause infection in others and children with a presumptive diagnosis of scalp ringworm should be treated with an imidazole cream whilst awaiting the results of mycological testing.

SCABIES

Diagnosis

Scabies is characterised by intense itching and a papular rash on the hands, genitalia and flexures. The diagnosis is confirmed by identification of the scabies burrow or run (**Figure 4.4**), which is a tiny raised linear white track

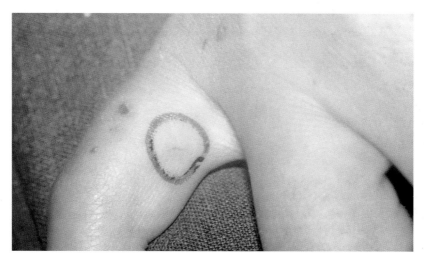

Figure 4.4 – Scabies burrow.

(1–4 mm long), typically occurring in the webs and along the sides of the fingers. The scabies mite (*Sarcoptes scabii*) lays its eggs in the burrow and its waste products lead to sensitisation and subsequent itch. This sensitisation takes about four weeks to develop.

Norwegian scabies

Patients with *Sarcoptes* infestation who are immunosuppressed (e.g. due to malnutrition, HIV or diabetes) are prone to an unpleasant, widespread, crusting and non-itchy form of the condition called Norwegian scabies. If immunosuppression is suspected, the urine should be checked for sugar and the patient referred for a medical opinion.

Treatment

Scabies is generally treated with an insecticide. The nurse prescriber can write malathion aqueous or alcoholic lotion or permethrin cream. Malathion is cheapest but has not been subjected to rigorous clinical trials. Random controlled trials suggest that permethrin cream is effective in 90% of cases (Walker and Johnstone, 1999) and this is currently the treatment of choice for patients over two years old. Scabicides should be applied to cool dry skin. Infected patients and their close contacts should be treated at the same time, regardless of whether they have symptoms or not. Box 4.2 summarises the treatment of scabies for the nurse prescriber.

The itch of scabies does not stop immediately after successful eradication treatment. The patient should be warned that the irritation might last two weeks or more. Since scabicides can themselves cause skin irritation, provided no new lesions appear, repeat treatment is unnecessary and undesirable.

Box 4.2 – Summary of NPF treatment for scabies

Available treatments	First Choice
	Permethrin 5% dermal cream. not recommended below 2 years
	Alternatives
	Malathion 0.5% aqueous lotion
	Malathion alcoholic lotion (not recommended due to skin irritation)

Box 4.2 – continued

Area to treat	Normal adults – whole body below the neck
	The elderly
	The immunosuppressed
	Children under 2 years } Whole body including head
	Treatment failures
How to apply?	To cool dry skin (not after a hot bath)
	Malathion lotion 24 hours
	Permethrin cream 8–12 hours
Review	After 10 days to check for new rash sites
Pruritus	Generally about 2 weeks (but may be longer)
Healing of lesions	Generally about 4 weeks
Who to treat?	Patient and all close contacts (in last 2 months)
Who to refer?	Infected scabies – needs antibiotics
	Norwegian (crusting) scabies – suggests immunosuppression
	Babies under 6 months

Head lice (Pediculosis)

Head lice are emotive little creatures; announcing their discovery requires delicacy and diplomacy. Head lice are common in primary school children and occur in the most regulated households; most parents are unbothered by the diagnosis but for some it may be a shock. A down-to-earth approach generally works best; parental anxiety can usually be calmed by emphasising the ease of treatment. Pruritus (itching) can take up to three months to develop consequently, most cases of head lice infestation are symptomless.

A letter from the head teacher, warning of an 'outbreak' of head lice at school, may provoke anxiety and psychosomatic head scratching. In such situations, beware of 'pseudo lice'. If careful detection combing of the family members does not reveal visible moving lice, reassurance would be more appropriate than the prophylactic use of insecticides.

Diagnosis

The presence of white or cream egg cases (nits) attached to the hairs is not, by itself, indicative of live louse infestation (**Figure 4.5**). Live head lice (*Pediculus humanus*) are grey or brown and can be difficult to spot whilst on the hair. They are, however, quite large (3–4 mm long) and can be easily seen if combed out onto a light surface.

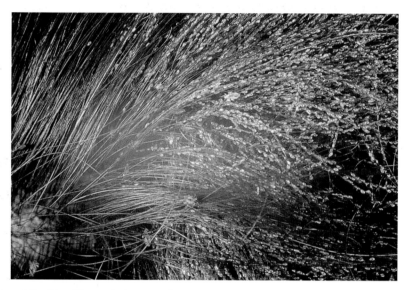

Figure 4.5 – Head lice and nits on scalp.

Secondary skin and scalp infections are common consequences of lice and scabies; these usually require treatment with antibiotics. In immunosuppressed individuals, these infections can be widespread and serious.

Practice Point

Patients who present with excoriation and an impetigo-like skin eruption should be checked for an infestation.

Treatment

Head lice treatments are summarised in Box 4.3. Concern about the potential harmful effects of insecticides has led to the withdrawal of some preparations (e.g. lindane) and warnings about others (e.g. carbaryl). In general, insecticides should be avoided where possible.

Box 4.3 – Summary of treatment of head lice

Available treatments	Malathion alcoholic lotion (not suitable in young children and patients with asthma or eczema)
	Malathion 0.5% aqueous lotion (suitable for all but may not be as effective as alcoholic lotion, and more likely to produce resistance)
	Permethrin 1% cream rinse
	Phenothrin 0.2% alcoholic lotion
	'Bug buster' combing treatment (no good-quality clinical trial evidence of effectiveness)
	Insecticide-containing shampoos (ineffective and not recommended)
	Tea tree oil and other herbal remedies (no published evidence of effectiveness, not recommended)
How to apply?	Malathion lotion – rub into dry hair, allow to dry, wash out after 12 hours
	Permethrin cream rinse – rub into damp hair, wash out after 10 minutes
	Phenothrin alcoholic lotion – rub in to dry hair, allow to dry, wash out after 2 hours
	Care must be taken not to apply insecticides directly to broken skin
Review	After 2–3 days detection combing to check for live lice
In case of treatment failure	Try an alternative treatment from the above list or refer to GP
Who needs detection combing?	All close contacts, family members, etc.

> **Box 4.3 – continued**
>
> Who to treat?   Only patients with LIVE LICE
>
> Who to refer?   Children under 6 months
>   Failure to clear after trying three insecticides (may need carbaryl which is not in the NPF)

Some people advocate 'bug buster' treatment protocols involving the application of conditioner and wet combing. Such 'environmentally friendly' regimens are appealing and inexpensive but their efficacy has not been proven by random controlled clinical trials (Dodd, 1999). Evidence is also lacking for the efficacy of herbal treatments. Clinical guidelines for the management of head lice infestation have been produced by many health authorities. The recommended treatment may reflect patterns of local insecticide resistance. Most now suggest that only patients that have visible 'live lice' (after combing) should receive insecticide treatments. Ask your local communicable disease department for a copy of guidelines applicable in your locality.

Shampoos are generally not effective in clearing head lice. Alcoholic solutions are useful for most adults and older children but they can induce skin irritation and bronchospasm; aqueous lotions should be used for babies and young children as well as people with asthma.

Other forms of lice

Body lice and crab lice are even more emotive than their scalp-borne cousins; they never fail to induce itching in healthcare professionals. Enquiries about lifestyle and sleeping arrangements are essential and shaving of infected areas and/or treatment of clothing may be desirable.

NAPPY RASH

Diagnosis

Nappy rash is generally due to irritation of the skin by urine and faeces and/or infection with *Candida* or bacteria. Uninfected irritant nappy rash tends to be confined to the nappy area and spares the flexures in the groin whereas *Candida* infection produces small red spots at the periphery of the nappy area (satellite lesions) and often spreads to the thighs.

Secondary bacterial infection should be suspected where there is severe inflammation or golden crusting (*impetigo*) present.

Management

The key to managing nappy rash is reduction of the irritation by urine and faeces and treatment of any secondary infection. Dramatic cures can usually be produced if the baby is nursed without nappies for a day or two. However, in the community, this is generally not practical.

Primary care management should be based on:

- good hygiene
- frequent nappy changes
- use of a topical antifungal preparation, if *Candida* is suspected
- use of a barrier preparation applied after every nappy change and over the topical antifungal
- referral for antibiotics, if bacterial infection is suspected.

The available literature suggests that there are no differences, of practical significance, between the various imidazole antifungal preparations in the NPF (clotrimazole 1% cream, econazole 1% cream and miconazole 2% cream). It would therefore be logical to start treatment with the cheapest.

CONSTIPATION

Constipation is a common complaint of the elderly and of parents about their children. Regular defaecation without pain or straining is important but daily evacuation is not essential if the patient is comfortable and the abdomen is not distended. Often reassurance of the patient or parent is possible if this normal variation is explained.

History

Appropriate questions to ask patients who complain of constipation are:

- How long has 'constipation' been a problem?
- How often do you have a bowel movement?
- Do you have to strain on defaecation?

- Are the stools hard?

- When did you last open your bowels?

The answers to the above questions should establish whether the patient has a real constipation problem.

- What medication are you taking?

Drug-induced causes of constipation are common.

- Have you felt nauseous or been sick?

- Do you have any abdominal pain?

A positive answer to one or both of these questions should raise suspicions of pathology.

- How much fluid do you drink each day?

Most adults need at least 8–10 cups.

Examination

The abdomen of a constipated patient should be examined to check for distension, tenderness, masses and colonic loading. For adults, a digital rectal examination would be appropriate to check for faecal loading.

Management

Many people complaining of constipation are not really constipated and many patients with constipation may be managed without prescribing a medicine (National Prescribing Centre, 1999a). Patients with sinister symptoms or signs (see Box 4.4) require referral.

Box 4.4 – Sinister symptoms/signs requiring referral

Vomiting

Abdominal pain/tenderness

Abdominal mass

Gaseous distension

Constipation alternating with diarrhoea

Blood or mucus in the stool

General advice to increase fluid and fibre intake is appropriate. However, important exceptions are those patients with impacted faeces or those who are particularly likely to become impacted (e.g. when opiates are prescribed). In such patients, high-fibre diets and bulking laxatives should be avoided because they can induce uncomfortable bloating and overflow of faeces.

Patients with sinister signs/symptoms should be discussed urgently with a GP. If the patients are on constipating drugs (National Prescribing Centre, 1999b), these should be reviewed by the original prescriber if possible.

Oral laxatives

Indications for prescribing laxatives are shown in Box 4.5. Most nurse prescribers will find that they can manage constipation using a few medicines. For most clinical situations, a bulk-forming laxative and a stimulant laxative (used individually or in combination) are effective (Passmore *et al*, 1993).

Box 4.5 – Indications for laxatives

Pain on defaecation or straining, during illness or pregnancy or after surgery

Frail elderly patients

In conjunction with constipating drugs (e.g. opiates)

Piles (haemorrhoids) or anal fissure

Bowel preparation for a diagnostic procedure (e.g. colonoscopy)

As part of a treatment of intestinal parasites.

Although lactulose is popular, it frequently causes uncomfortable flatulence (Kot and Pettit-Young, 1992) and is not as effective as a combination of a bulking and a stimulant laxative (Passmore *et al*, 1993).

There appears to be no reliable clinical trial evidence comparing the efficacy of the various laxative classes (bulk forming, stimulant and osmotic) (Tramonte *et al*, 1997).

Enemas and suppositories

In the absence of sinister symptoms or signs, faecal impaction or loading generally requires use of laxative suppositories or enemas.

Biochemical disturbances can be induced by the regular use of enemas in debilitated patients. Periodic biochemical (blood) monitoring would be appropriate in such cases.

Constipation in babies and children

Symptoms and signs of constipation in childhood are numerous and may include a poor appetite, lack of energy, behaviour changes, pain or bleeding on defaecation and soiling (Muir, 1999). Enemas or suppositories should not be prescribed by nurses for babies or children. They are rarely needed, even in hospital practice, and they can be psychologically traumatising.

Oral laxatives are not generally required for children or babies. In constipated children who are otherwise well, masterly inactivity and confident reassurance is generally the best regimen to adopt. Advise the parent about fluids and fibre intake and wait; some children may take over a week to have a bowel movement.

Constipation in infants should be taken seriously and generally warrants referral to exclude bowel obstruction, cerebral palsy or Hirschsprung's disease.

THREADWORMS

Diagnosis

Threadworms usually present with itching around the anus leading to scratching. Sometimes, there are signs of excoriation of the anal skin. In most cases, the infection is not serious, although rarely complications can occur (National Prescribing Centre, 1999c). Threadworms are common in children at primary school but can affect all ages. The worms look like small threads of white cotton and may be seen on the faeces or round the anus. They emerge from the bowel onto the perianal skin at night, to lay their eggs. Threadworms can be identified by applying a piece of Sellotape, sticky side down, to the perianal area before rising in the morning and then examining the tape against a dark background.

In most cases, it is desirable to identify the threadworm prior to initiating treatment. However, in cases where the history leads to a high index of suspicion or when another member of the household is infected, it may be appropriate to begin treating people even when worms have not been seen.

Management

Threadworms and their eggs may stick under the fingernails and can contaminate clothing, bedclothes, flannels and towels. Spread of infection and reinfection of the host may be prevented by scrupulous hygiene (National Prescribing Centre, 1999c) to prevent the recycling of eggs from anus to mouth.

There are no robust trials comparing currently available treatments for threadworms but limited evidence suggests the preparations in the NPF have comparable efficacy. The age of the patient and the simplicity of the dosage regimen is one method that can be used to determine an effective treatment (see Box 4.6).

Box 4.6 – Treatment of threadworms

Treatments	First Choice – Mebendazole A single dose Not licensed for children under 2
	Second Choice – Piperazine and senna powder (Pripsen) Repeat dose after 14 days Licensed for children from 3 months
	Note cautions in NPF
Other measures	Wash hands before meals and after using lavatory Keep nails short and avoid putting hands in mouth Bathe or shower in morning Avoid sharing towels/flannels Change bedlinen and nightwear as frequently as is practical
In case of recurrence	Repeat treatment and refer if infection persists
Who to treat?	Whole household
Who to refer?	Pregnant females If infection is persistent

BOILS AND CARBUNCLES

A boil is caused by bacterial infection of a hair follicle with the subsequent accumulation of pus. A carbuncle is a collection of several boils that have merged.

Incision and drainage

Left to their own devices, most boils build up pus, 'point' and burst to the skin surface. A pointing boil can be very tender but once discharge has started, the pain diminishes and it begins to heal.

Many nurses will feel happy to lance a pointing boil. A quick 'slash' with a scalpel blade generally does the trick and the procedure can be performed without local anaesthetic. The incision must be of sufficient size to facilitate good drainage of pus. A hypodermic needle is not a suitable instrument for lancing boils.

It is generally not a good idea to squeeze a discharging boil as this can push infection into surrounding tissues.

Magnesium sulphate paste

The application of a magnesium sulphate paste dressing is a tried and tested treatment for a boil. Magnesium sulphate paste should be prescribed with appropriate absorbent dressing material and adhesive tape (e.g. sterile gauze and Micropore® tape). The paste should be stirred and applied thickly to the dressing material which should be changed every day. Running warm water over the boil prior to redressing helps to increase blood supply to the region and promote drainage and healing.

Antibiotics

Generally, antibiotics are not required for simple boils. Antibiotics turn the pus of a boil into a sterile collection of fluid that can remain unabsorbed for weeks.

Boils or other skin infections in the so-called 'danger area' of the face (**Figure 4.6**) are an exception to the above advice and antibiotics should be used in such cases. The anatomy of the blood vessels in this region is such that a bacterial infection may spread to the brain and develop into a potentially fatal cavernous sinus thrombosis.

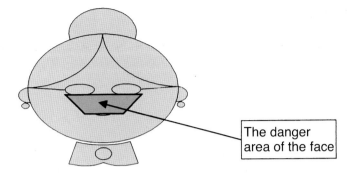

Figure 4.6 – The 'danger area' of the face.

Carbuncles are multiloculated and cannot be readily treated by a simple incision or magnesium sulphate paste dressings. They generally require systemic antibiotics.

Diabetes and bacterial carriers

Patients with recurrent boils or carbuncles may have diabetes or persistent skin carriage. The urine from all patients with boils should be checked for glucose. Some patients carry boil-causing bacteria (*Staphylococcus aureus*) on their skin and up their noses. Pathological skin bacteria can be eliminated by the use of an antiseptic skin wash such as chlorhexidine (not in the NPF). Nasal carriage may require an antiseptic or antibiotic nasal cream such as Naseptin (not in the NPF).

ORAL THRUSH

Diagnosis

Candida albicans is a yeast-like plant that is present in the normal digestive tract. It is not normally troublesome or visible. Overgrowth of *Candida* (thrush) is common in babies and women. Generally, growth of the organism in the mouth (**Figure 4.7**) or in the genital region is suggestive of a change in the local environment. Extensive oral thrush would merit referral for further investigation.

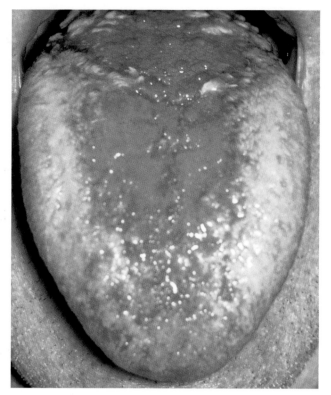

Figure 4.7 – *Candida* of tongue.

Oral thrush is commonly seen in infants as a milk-like deposit around the gums or tongue. However, unlike milk, the deposit of *Candida* cannot be scraped away with a tongue depressor. Thrush can be passed between babies and breast-feeding mothers and leads to intense pain or cracking of the nipples.

In adults, oral thrush may be associated with the use of steroid inhalers or it may occur in immunosuppressed individuals (e.g. diabetes, cancer or HIV). The urine of such individuals should be checked for glucose. Mouth rinsing should be encouraged in patients using steroid inhalers.

Management

Treatments for oral thrush work on contact with the yeast. They should be used after meals and should be retained in the mouth as long as possible. The NPF has two preparations for oral thrush (see Box 4.7).

Superficial thrush of the nipples in breast-feeding mothers may be treated by applying miconazole cream to the nipple after each feed. The baby should be treated as above even if symptoms are only noticed in the mother. If *Candida* has entered the milk ducts, breast pain is deep seated and oral treatment is required (not currently in the NPF).

Box 4.7 – Management of oral thrush	
Nystatin	Available as: oral suspension – for babies and young children pastilles – for adults
Miconazole gel	Although this is more expensive, it generally clears thrush more quickly than Nystatin suspension

EAR WAX

Ear wax is a natural lubricant secreted by glands within the ear canal. This canal is self-cleaning with thousands of tiny hair-like cilia wafting foreign bodies (and wax) outwards.

Ears do not require regular cleaning and patients – and their parents – should be discouraged from using cotton buds, match sticks, hair grips, pencils or any other probes for removing wax. Blind probing invariably compacts the wax and can injure the canal wall, the ciliary 'escalator' or the eardrum.

Diagnosis and management of ear wax is straightforward in all patients without previous ear disease. Accumulation of ear wax is the most common cause of deafness. Often the deafness occurs acutely when the last part of the ear canal becomes blocked (e.g. with water following a shower or swim).

History

Two aspects of the history are important when wax blockage is suspected.

- Is there any history of previous ear disease?

In patients who have had previous ear disease, where other pathology is suspected, referral may be appropriate even if wax is present.

- Is there any pain?

Wax does not generally cause pain and painful ears should generally not be syringed.

Examination

When examining the ear, make sure you have an auriscope with a good light. Most modern instruments use a halogen bulb with a magnifying lens and should provide an excellent view, but 'treatment room' instruments are sometimes not well cared for. Occasionally the battery is flat, the light is incorrectly directed or the specula have been lost. A medium–sized speculum is appropriate to use in most cases. If the ear canal is gently straightened, by pulling the ear lobe (*pinna*) backwards, one should be able to obtain a clear view of the eardrum (*tympanic membrane*) and identify some important landmarks such as the malleus handle and the 'cone of light'(**Figure 4.8**).

Although the principles of using an auriscope are not difficult to learn, the interpretation of what you see may take longer. For the nurse prescriber, the most important part of examination is to identify wax blocking the ear canal. Wax may appear grey or brown. It may be hard and dry or greasy and soft. A white, yellow or green liquid discharge suggests the presence of pus (and infection). A coal-black deposit in the ear canal is suggestive of a fungus infection (*Aspergillus nigra*). It is not necessary to diagnose the cause of an abnormal eardrum but it is useful to be able to recognise deviation from normality.

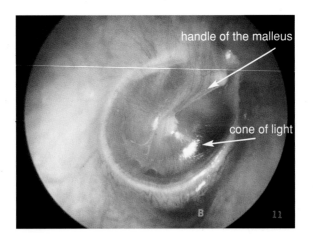

Figure 4.8 – Normal right eardrum as seen through an auriscope.

Management

A number of OTC preparations are available for softening ear wax. Some contain powerful organic solvents which, although undoubtedly effective, can cause irritation to the external ear canal.

The NPF has two preparations for softening wax (olive oil and almond oil). There would seem to be no evidence in the literature that one of these is more effective than the other. It is not necessary to warm the oil before insertion, nor should cotton wool be inserted, but the patient should be advised to lie down for a few minutes with the affected ear uppermost to allow the drops to run into the wax. After softening, some wax will clear spontaneously with the aid of the ciliary escalator.

However, some adult patients will require syringing. Effective and safe ear syringing is a useful skill that is easily learnt within primary care. Perforation of the eardrum can occur if excessive water pressure is used for syringing ears. The risk of perforation can be reduced by using one of the modern pulsed water devices rather than a traditional 'icing syringe'. Patients are usually extremely grateful to have their hearing restored. Don't forget to check that you can see the normal eardrum after completion of ear syringing.

References

Dodd, C.S. (1999). Interventions for treating head lice. *Cochrane Library*, vol. 3.

Kot, T.V. & Pettit-Young, N.A. (1992). Lactulose in the management of constipation: a current review. *Annals of Pharmacotherapy* 26:1277–1282.

Marks, R. (1993). *Roxburgh's Common Skin Diseases*. London: Chapman and Hall Medical.

Mehta, D.K. (ed.) (2000). *The British National Formulary 40*. London: British Medical Association and Royal Pharmaceutical Society of Great Britain.

Muir, J. (1999). *Guidelines for the Management of Childhood Constipation*. Medical Information Unit, Hull: Reckitt and Colman Products.

National Prescribing Centre (1999a). Dietary fibre in the management of constipation. Prescribing Nurse Fact Sheet No. 16, September.

National Prescribing Centre (1999b). The management of constipation. Prescribing Nurse Bulletin Vol. 1, No. 6.

National Prescribing Centre (1999c). The management of scabies and threadworms. Prescribing Nurse Bulletin Vol. l, No. 3.

Passmore, A.P., Wilson-Davies, K., Stoker, C., Scott, M. E. (1993). Chronic constipation in long stay elderly patients: a comparison of lactulose and a senna-fibre combination. *British Medical Journal* 307:769–771.

Rudikoff, D. & Lebwohl, M. (1998). Atopic dermatitis. *Lancet* 351:1715–1721.

Tramonte, S.M., Brand, M.B., Mulrow, C.D., Amato, M.G., O'Keefe, M.E., Ramirez, G. (1997). The treatment of chronic constipation in adults: a systematic review. *Journal of General Internal Medicine* 12: 15–24.

Walker, G.J.A. & Johnstone, P.W. (1999). Interventions for treating scabies. *Cochrane Library*, vol. 3.

5

CURRENT ISSUES IN NURSE PRESCRIBING: A PHARMACIST'S PERSPECTIVE

A clear and consistent message from evaluations of the nurse-prescribing demonstration sites is that the introduction of nurse prescribing has had a beneficial effect on relationships between community/practice nurses and pharmacists. Nurses are keen to access practical help and support on prescribing issues and pharmacists generally enjoy sharing their specific expertise about medication with appreciative colleagues. In addition, both groups may be aware that the advent of nurse prescribing offers an unparalleled opportunity to start with a 'clean sheet' and improve prescribing practices.

This chapter looks at:

1. how pharmacists can support nurse prescribers

2. sources of drug information for nurse prescribers

3. after implementation – the pharmacy issues:

   - nurse prescribing or supply under a group protocol

   - to bulk purchase or not, particularly dressings

- relationships with the pharmaceutical industry

- developing prescribing guidelines or formularies

4. financial issues and monitoring of nurse prescribing:

  - how nurse-prescribing budgets are set

  - monitoring nurse-prescribing expenditure

  - how to link with general practitioner (GP) prescribing of Nurse Prescribers' Formulary NPF items

  - early results from nurse-prescribing pilot sites

  - issues for primary care groups (PCG/Ts) and primary care trusts (PCTs).

HOW PHARMACISTS CAN SUPPORT NURSE PRESCRIBERS

Prescribing nurses may come into contact with a number of pharmacists, each practising in a different environment.

Community pharmacists

Community pharmacists dispense most prescriptions written by nurse prescribers (unless for patients in rural areas who receive medicines from a dispensing practice) and have a natural interest in developing good working relationships with local health professionals. Many community pharmacists are actively participating in PCGs and local stakeholder meetings may provide ideal opportunities to discuss issues of mutual interest such as wound management guidelines. Many community pharmacists are making a useful contribution to local updates and seminars for nurse prescribers, on both a formal and informal basis.

Health authority pharmaceutical advisers

The role of health authority pharmaceutical advisers, like that of health authorities (HAs), is changing significantly. They have traditionally been responsible for setting GP prescribing budgets, working with GPs to improve prescribing practice and managing the HA prescribing agenda. As their role has widened and increased in complexity, many have gained experience in developing prescribing strategies and advising on priorities for the use of drug treatment. They are often in a position to draw on their experience with local GPs to advise nurse prescribers, although their responsibilities will change to reflect the more strategic role that HAs will have in the future. Establishing mechanisms for managing the introduction of new drugs to the NHS and leading the development of clinical governance in local health communities will continue to be important HA responsibilities.

Community trust/community services pharmacists

These pharmacists work for NHS trusts and their role includes the provision of pharmacy support and supply of stock medication to local community health service staff. They may be involved in the provision of specific education and training and drug information for nurse prescribers. As they may work alongside community nurse trust colleagues, they often provide practical support to the nurse-prescribing implementation programme, e.g. security issues, ordering of prescription pads and monitoring expenditure at trust level.

Primary care group/trust pharmaceutical advisers

This new group of pharmacists are rapidly establishing themselves at a local level and many new nurse prescribers will have already made contact with them. PCG/T/PCT pharmaceutical advisers are taking on some of the roles formerly carried out by advisers in HAs, including budget setting at practice level and monitoring and reporting on GP prescribing expenditure.

Nurse prescribers will need to get to know all these pharmacists locally and, as will be seen later in this chapter, they will have to work in close collaboration in order to monitor prescribing within the NPF effectively.

Pharmacists act as tutors for part of the taught programme for nurse prescribing, both for Mode 1 students, i.e. qualified community nurses holding a district nursing (DN) or health visiting (HV) qualification, and Mode 2 students, i.e. nurses undertaking specialist community practitioner programmes (see Chapter 1). They may also provide local support sessions for nurses either during or after they have completed training.

In many areas, nurses are actively encouraged to visit local community pharmacies to see at first hand how the dispensing process is managed. This provides an ideal opportunity to explore problem areas and how nurse prescribing will affect each other's future roles. Community pharmacists will be keen to know how they can contact nurses if queries arise on prescriptions and nurses need to familiarise themselves with common pack sizes and pitfalls in prescription writing.

Community nurse managers and trust pharmacists will consider the practical aspects of implementation such as administrative support, establishing safe systems for prescription pads (classified as controlled stationery), revising job descriptions to include nurse prescribing and negotiation with the HA on the initial budget for nurse prescribing by trust employees.

Sources of drug information for nurse prescribers

The centrally provided key references for nurse prescribers include:

- British National Formulary (BNF), including the NPF
- Drug Tariff
- bulletins and factsheets from the National Prescribing Centre.

In addition, the following may be of interest.

Drug information centres (now renamed medicines information centres)

These are located within some NHS trust pharmacy departments and also at regional centres. They are able to answer enquiries and also provide a range of bulletins.

Internet websites

The National Prescribing Centre's website at *www.npc.co.uk* includes a section specifically for nurse prescribers. Some drug information centres now have websites, which provide an ideal way to access updated information. The site developed by the South Thames Drug Information Centre is an excellent example at *www.druginfozone.org*

Product literature from the pharmaceutical industry

The back of the BNF includes a listing of telephone numbers for most major companies and nurses will receive increasing amounts of direct mail. Helplines relating to specific products are also available. Some of these resources are extremely useful but nurse prescribers will need to develop critical appraisal skills if they are to effectively evaluate the literature. Many pharmacists have well-developed appraisal skills and can advise nurses or contribute through teaching sessions.

Pharmacy professionals

People who can be contacted for drug information include the following.

- *Community pharmacists* are keen to support nurse prescribers and are the most accessible source of practical product information. New nurse prescribers would be well advised to proactively visit their local pharmacies.

- *Pharmacists in trusts, HA and PCG/T/PCTs* may all be able to help nurses with specific queries within their areas of expertise. For instance, enquiries about budget issues or product choice within formularies may be referred to PCG/T/PCT or HA pharmaceutical advisers. Trust pharmacists can help with clinical or organisational queries, e.g. information on vaccines, trust clinical guidelines or procedures.

- *Specialist nurse or pharmacist colleagues* are available locally and usually their role includes advice and support to other practitioners. These may include continence nurse specialists, tissue viability nurses, care of the elderly specialist nurses and pharmacists, and directorate pharmacists covering specialities such as paediatrics, HIV and AIDs or community liaison.

AFTER IMPLEMENTATION – THE PHARMACY ISSUES

As the implementation phase of nurse prescribing is so demanding, it can be difficult to focus attention adequately on the issues which will arise once significant numbers of nurses are prescribing. It will not take very long, however, for this to change and this section considers some important issues which need to be considered in the medium and longer term. Nurse prescribing is only one of a number of recent developments affecting prescribing, some of these developments being linked. Prescribing nurses will increasingly need to understand the relevance of each topic to their practice. Key areas concerning medication and prescribing are highlighted below.

Nurse prescribing or supply under a group protocol (recently renamed patient group directions (PGD)

There has been widespread confusion about the definition of these terms. The definitions given in the final report of the Crown Review Group Department of Health (DoH, 1999) are as follows.

Nurse prescribing:

'Community nurse or practice nurse who is identified as a nurse prescriber on the UKCC register, writing a prescription for an item in the Nurse Prescribers' Formulary using form FP10 (CN) or FP10 (PN), within a nurse prescribing demonstration scheme or within a Health Authority or Trust that has implemented nurse prescribing.'

Patient Group Direction (PGD) (formerly Group Protocol):

'A Patient Group Direction is a specific written instruction for the supply and administration, or administration of a named medicine in an identified clinical situation. It applies to groups of patients who may not be individually identified before presenting for treatment. PGDs are drawn up locally by doctors, pharmacists and other health professionals, signed by a doctor or dentist and a pharmacist as appropriate, and approved by an appropriate healthcare body.'

Patient-specific written directions:

'A written statement defining the management of a named patient which has been agreed by the doctor and nurse responsible for the patient, and by any other appropriate health professionals.'

Why is there confusion over these definitions? Some initiatives (particularly in hospital trusts) have been referred to as 'nurse prescribing' when in fact nurses are issuing or administering medicines under a group protocol/PGD of some description. Also, it is sometimes quite difficult to decide whether certain protocols operating in the community are PGDs or 'patient-specific' protocols, as they may contain elements of both types. The key issues are that nurses who prescribe (although from a limited formulary) are acting independently in assessing their patients' needs and are not restricted to a predefined clinical situation. In contrast, PGDs/group protocols are intended to cover the more predictable situations in which medicines may need to be supplied or administered, such as immunisation or contraception. The position on patient-specific written directions, where for instance, doses of insulin or pain relief may be altered, is less clear and further central guidance is awaited.

In August 2000, new regulations were approved and the NHS Executive issued Health Services Circular 2000/026 which gives definitive guidance on Patient Group Directions (PGD). All PGDs must now comply with the new legal requirements, which cover how they are drawn up, and arrangements for security, storage and labelling of the medicines involved. Guidance is also given on the circumstances in which antibiotics and black triangle drugs may be included.

In this new era, nurse prescribers may be faced with a choice between writing a prescription or supplying or administering a medicine under a PGD/group protocol. It may be helpful to consider both the advantages and disadvantages of each option and an analysis of the strengths, weaknesses, opportunities and threats for each option can prove to be a valuable exercise within a staff team.

Box 5.1 – Advantages and disadvantages of nurse prescribing

Advantages of nurse prescribing	*Disadvantages of nurse prescribing*
Nurses act as independent prescribers and make own decisions on diagnosis and treatment	Possibility of inconsistent prescribing across different professional groups
Eligible nurses can prescribe for a GP's patients in any community setting	Prescribing only from restricted formulary
Opportunity to strengthen links with local pharmacists	Difficulties with cross-HA border prescribing, homeless people and nurse-led clinics e.g. leg ulcer treatment
All prescribing data captured automatically through prescription pricing authority (PPA) prescription analysis and cost trends (PACT) reports and easily available for audit	Complex monitoring requirement to review prescribing by both nurses and GPs from NPF

Box 5.1 – *continued*

Advantages of nurse prescribing	*Disadvantages of nurse prescribing*
No stockholding necessary for community nurses – full range of products accessible from community pharmacies, including weekends	Depends on adequate stocks within community pharmacies and ability of patient to visit pharmacy
Reduces waste as prescriptions can be written as often as necessary	Greater budgetary risks for service managers
Promotes greater integration of prescribing practice with medical staff	Potential to create tensions with medical staff around clinical and financial issues
	No plans yet to allow nurse prescribing via practice computer systems

Box 5.2 – Advantages and disadvantages of supply under PDG/group protocol (this will vary slightly for <u>administration, c.f. supply</u>, under PDG/group protocol)

Advantages	*Disadvantages*
'One stop' treatment – patient receives medication without delay	Supply can only operate in defined settings such as minor injuries units (but generally not GP practices)
Few restrictions on range of treatments that can be included – only controlled drugs (CDs) and black triangle drugs (where the Committee for Safety of Medicines requires special monitoring) are discouraged or excluded	Restricted to predefined clinical circumstances – difficult to respond if unpredicted needs arise

---

Box 5.2 – continued

Advantages	Disadvantages
Control over presentation and labelling of products supplied	Additional workload of purchase and stockholding of prepacked and prelabelled medication
Group protocol gives detailed clinical framework for practitioner	Little scope for individual clinical judgements due to legal constraints
Promotes consistent prescribing practice, regardless of practitioner	No second person check on accuracy of supply/dispensing process
Endorsement of protocol by medical practitioners is required	Huge workload in preparation, implementation and training associated with new group protocol
	Loss of routine patient contact with community pharmacist for advice and information
	Opposition from community pharmacists if reduces dispensing income

---

To bulk purchase or not, particularly dressings

Service managers may also be asked to consider schemes whereby instead of writing FP10 (CN) prescriptions for items such as wound dressings, the trust (or PCT) purchases in bulk and nurses supply these items to patients from a bulk stock. This arrangement has been trialled in some trusts and has provoked considerable interest, but also an equal measure of concern. This is a far-reaching decision, which will impact on many other agencies including community pharmacies and patients, so careful consideration needs to be taken of all the potential effects. A useful way forward would be to host a stakeholder meeting involving nurses, practice staff, GPs and pharmacists, in which a full analysis is carried out. Box 5.3 highlights some of the advantages and disadvantages of bulk purchase of dressing products for use by community nurses.

Box 5.3 – Advantages and disadvantages of bulk purchase of dressing products for use by community nurses

Advantages	Disadvantages
Cost savings through contracts with supplying companies	Likely decrease in cost saving year on year
A supply always available to any nurse in an emergency (not just nurse prescribers)	Data on supply and use of dressing products no longer automatically available through PACT reports
Immediate supply available without delay, e.g. for housebound patients	An ordering and distribution system will need to be set up and fully costed
May be of particular value for dressing packs (for nurse rather than patient use)	Central and local storage facilities will be needed
Can include products not available in the drug tariff, if funding sufficient	Access to store may be limited at weekends and evenings
	Relationships with local community pharmacists may be adversely affected
	Only a limited range of dressing products likely to be available in bulk; others will require FP10 prescription

Both PGDs and possible bulk purchasing of products illustrate very well the need for nurses to consult widely with colleagues and patients when considering future options. It may be very tempting to go for options which promise cost savings in the short term but may bring wider disadvantages when the effect on the whole health system is taken into account.

Relationships with the pharmaceutical industry

Workshops held for recently qualified nurse prescribers have frequently highlighted concerns about future relationships with pharmaceutical industry representatives. There may be very different approaches operating at practice level, with some GPs rarely seeing representatives and others hosting regular industry-sponsored 'drug lunches'. There is a need for all organisations and practitioners to agree locally consistent practices. This can be achieved through initiatives led by the HA or PCG/T. Since PCG/Ts are subcommittees of HAs, any HA policy on industry relationships will apply equally to them. The policy will need to address activities of representatives, samples and free gifts, sponsorship of meetings or educational activities and promotional materials. This is a good topic for discussion at multidisciplinary PCG/T meetings and is likely to provoke lively debate.

Developing prescribing guidelines or formularies

The implementation of nurse prescribing has necessitated formulary development or the development of guidelines in key therapeutic areas. These areas include wound management, the treatment for head lice and scabies, and emollients. The development of guidelines can produce tensions between trusts, PCG/Ts and individual practices over who 'controls' prescribing practice. This needs to be sensitively managed. GPs will need to be reassured that some controls or guidelines are in place for nurses that they do not directly employ, while trusts will naturally have concerns over nurse prescribing expenditure for which they are held accountable. It would seem desirable for trusts to work jointly with PCG/Ts on prescribing guidelines but to leave formulary development to PCG/Ts and practices. This distinction needs to be made since guidelines define good practice, whereas formularies are intended to be restrictive and are most effective if agreed at a very local level.

FINANCIAL ISSUES AND MONITORING OF NURSE PRESCRIBING

How nurse-prescribing budgets are set

As initially there was a lack of accurate historical data on which to base budget setting, the majority of HAs drew upon the experience at Bolton and other pilot sites and allocated 1% of the primary care prescribing budget. What this means is that out of the total sum available for prescribing by GPs within a HA, 1% has been set aside as a notional budget for nurse prescribing and the community trust, as budget holder, is accountable for expenditure. It is important to appreciate that there is no new money available for nurse prescribing. Instead of asking a GP to sign a prescription on their behalf, nurse prescribers are able to do this themselves. It is anticipated that there will be no greater demand on prescribing resource than before and that prescribing by nurses is, in effect, substituting what was previously done by GPs.

This formula has generally worked well, as long as trusts do not provide any dressings or other products to patients via their hospital stores. In the latter case, if nurses now prescribe all these, this may lead to budget problems. For example, if most items used by DNs were prescribed by GPs but now the nurse is able to prescribe them for herself, there is no practical difference in the overall primary care prescribing allocation. However, if most of the DN items have been historically supplied through a hospital stores, the effect of nurse prescribing is to put additional pressure on the primary care prescribing allocation. It was evident from pilot sites that, by the end of the first year, the nurse-prescribing budget was underspent. This was primarily due to the time taken for nurses to complete their courses, become eligible as prescribers and to receive their prescription pads. In the second year, it was identified that the budget had been overspent due to an insufficient top-slice. Now in the third year, after a 1% top-slice with only seven months data available, the budget looks like it will break even (this information was gained at DoH pilot project meetings).

From April 1999, with the formation of PCG/Ts which are subcommittees of their respective HA, nurse-prescribing budgets fell within an overall cash-limited prescribing budget. In practice, this means that overspending in prescribing directly impacts upon the budget for secondary care. The concept of firm cash limits on prescribing is new to primary care and poses a considerable challenge to the newly formed PCG/Ts. Therefore, all prescribers must have a heightened awareness of their prescribing costs and be able to make informed decisions, which promote clinically effective and cost-effective prescribing.

Monitoring nurse-prescribing expenditure

The community trust is responsible for monitoring how the budget for nurse prescribing is spent through information received in the form of PACT reports from the PPA. There are different reports available. A full PACT catalogue provides the full prescribing data on every nurse within a trust by item and cost. For budget-monitoring purposes, there is a report for each trust which provides the spend per month against budget and projects the over/underspend based on the cumulative monthly spend.

The budget-monitoring statement is useful in that it provides in-year predictions of under/overspend. For clinical governance, though, the full PACT catalogue is of greater value as this can be used to assess adherence to local guidelines or protocols and can highlight prescribing behaviour which is out of step with colleagues carrying similar caseloads.

Individual nurse prescribers should receive a PACT catalogue detailing their own prescribing on a regular basis. In many trusts, the effort involved in providing this is perhaps far greater than expected. Currently, each trust receives one full PACT catalogue monthly showing all prescribing by nurses employed within the trust. Photocopying and distributing each individual's copy is a significant burden for a trust employing a large number of nurses. The development of electronic PACT data (ePACT) can make the data more accessible and provide the means of obtaining comparative data which may be more useful and meaningful to nurses than a catalogue of their own prescribing. Trusts need to consider who is best able to manipulate the data to provide regular reports as well as carrying out an assessment of what nurse prescribers themselves would find most valuable. Over a period of 10 years or so, GP PACT data has developed into a valuable monitoring tool enabling comparisons within both a HA area and nationally. These data can readily identify practices with above or below average prescribing for that HA in any major BNF category (cardiovascular, gastrointestinal, central nervous system, etc.) and serve to focus the attention of medical and pharmaceutical advisers on individuals and practices as part of their monitoring role.

Nurse managers will wish to monitor prescribing data to ensure adherence to local treatment protocols or clinical guidelines, as part of the trust's clinical governance agenda. From the financial perspective, nurse managers and PCG/Ts will be keen to monitor prescribing against budget. This is particularly high on PCG/Ts' agendas because any further call on primary care prescribing budgets within an overall cash-limited budget allows much less flexibility for primary care developments.

How to link with GP expenditure of NPF items

It is possible to produce PACT reports detailing expenditure by GP practice on NPF items. This is important to monitor because the expected trend is for GP prescribing of NPF items to fall once nurse prescribing is up and running. If it doesn't fall, it may indicate difficulties within the practice, such as a disagreement over new working arrangements. The nurse prescriber may need help to resolve such difficulties. Where a

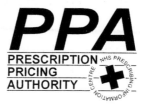

PRESCRIBING	
MONITORING	
DOCUMENT	

**PRESCRIPTION
PRICING
AUTHORITY**

Report to:

> **Dr WORKLOAD**
> **47 BRONCHODILATOR WAY**
> **MYOCARDIAL INFARCATION**
> **REFLUXSHIRE**
>
>
> **NSA 1DS**

For more information contact:
Help Desk, Prescription Pricing Authority, Block B, Scottish Life House, Archbold Terrace, Jesmond, Newcastle-upon-Tyne, NE2 1DB.
Telephone: (0191) 2035050 Fax: (0191) 2035001

Figure 5.1 – Sample page from PACT catalogue.

Prescription Pricing Authority

Community Unit Contract Practice Summary Sheet

Prescribing Monitoring Document (Actual Cost)

For the month of September 1999

WORKLOAD NHS TRUST

An asterisk next to the practice code denotes a Personal Medical Services (PMS) Pilot.
This statement relates to prescriptions dispensed in September 1999

WARNING The figures shown on this report are for monitoring purposes only and do not reflect the actual charge to the cash limit.

Practice Code	Name	Monthly Actual Cost £	Cumul. Actual Cost £
522023	Dr WORKLOAD THE SURGERY 01 ANON ROAD	5	5
522034	Dr WORKLOAD THE SURGERY 02 ANON ROAD	0	0
542014	Dr WORKLOAD THE SURGERY 03 ANON ROAD	0	17
542032	Dr WORKLOAD THE SURGERY 04 ANON ROAD	0	80
582003	Dr WORKLOAD THE SURGERY 05 ANON ROAD	0	2
582005	Dr WORKLOAD THE SURGERY 06 ANON ROAD	0	5
582006	Dr WORKLOAD THE SURGERY 07 ANON ROAD	0	30
582007	Dr WORKLOAD THE SURGERY 08 ANON ROAD	0	7
582015	Dr WORKLOAD THE SURGERY 09 ANON ROAD	0	24
582016	Dr WORKLOAD THE SURGERY 10 ANON ROAD	0	0

Page 1

FRP530

#00001/00002/06-04-2000/004293521/

Figure 5.2 – Sample page from PACT catalogue.

practice nurse is a prescriber, the practice PACT data will show a figure for this expenditure but it will not be possible from the practice report to see the breakdown by product.

Early results from nurse-prescribing pilot site

In East Kent at least, GPs' initial fears about nurses prescribing more paracetamol and head lice lotions have not been realised. Evidence suggests that DNs have not been persuaded by pharmaceutical industry hype about new dressings and the budget has not been exceeded.

Issues for PCGs and PCTs

In some regions a nurse prescribing clinical and financial governance group meets regularly to review expenditure against budget and is involved in the development of clinical guidelines and the future training needs for nurse prescribers. As dressings constitute the largest area of spend in some areas, separate wound management groups have been established to review the clinical management of leg ulcers and dressings choices, with the development of 'best buy' product guides. Drawing on nurse prescribers' expertise, formularies for GP practices, identifying wound care strategies when assessing patients in nursing homes, have also been developed.

Future challenges for nurse prescribing are likely to be both financial and clinical. Issues to consider include the following.

- What happens if the budget is overspent? A contingency may be held at the PCG/T to cover overspending by GPs. However, will trusts have to cut services, delay purchasing equipment or leave vacancies unfilled to make up a shortfall at the year end?

- What happens if the budget is underspent? Will the underspend be kept by the Trust or the HA? Alternatively, will it be returned to the PCG/T to offset any GP overspending or to pay for prescribing incentive schemes?

- How will new products be managed?

- Who will arbitrate if there is a difference of opinion about a move to a central purchasing policy?

- How do we know that evidence-based treatments are being used?

- What outcome data are available?

#00001/00002/07-04-2000/003975065

CONTENTS

This report consists of a Catalogue of Prescribing (full).

Prescribing details are shown in the following BNF classifications as requested:

01	Gastro-Intestinal System			
02	Cardiovascular System	***	no prescribing	***
03	Respiratory System	***	no prescribing	***
04	Central Nervous System			
05	Infections			
06	Endocrine System			
07	Obstetrics,Gynae+Urinary Tract Disorders			
08	Malignant Disease & Immunosuppression	***	no prescribing	***
09	Nutrition And Blood			
10	Musculoskeletal & Joint Diseases	***	no prescribing	***
11	Eye	***	no prescribing	***
12	Ear, Nose And Oropharynx			
13	Skin			
14	Immunological Products & Vaccines	***	no prescribing	***
15	Anaesthesia			
18	Preparations used in Diagnosis	***	no prescribing	***
19	Other Drugs And Preparations			
20	Dressings			
21	Appliances			
22	Incontinence Appliances			
23	Stoma Appliances			

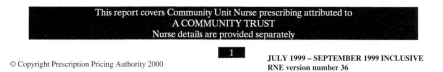

This report covers Community Unit Nurse prescribing attributed to
A COMMUNITY TRUST
Nurse details are provided separately

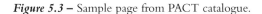

© Copyright Prescription Pricing Authority 2000

JULY 1999 – SEPTEMBER 1999 INCLUSIVE
RNE version number 36

Figure 5.3 – Sample page from PACT catalogue.

CATALOGUE OF PRESCRIBING (full)

#00001/00003/07-04-2000/00397506.

UNIDENTIFIED PATIENT PRACTICE Quantity

	No. of Items	Quantity x Items	Cost(£)

00A0001E NR WORKLOAD

5. Infections

5.2 Antifungal Drugs

5.2.0 Antifungal Drugs

	Quantity	No. of Items	Quantity x Items	Cost(£)
Nystatin Oral Susp 100,000u/ml	30	1	30	2.20
		1	30	2.20
Sub-total Nystatin (Systemic)		1		2.20
Sub-total Chem. Sub. Nystatin		1		2.20
Sub-total 5.2.0		1		2.20
SUB-TOTAL 5.2		1		2.20
Total: Infections		1		2.20

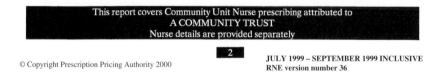

This report covers Community Unit Nurse prescribing attributed to
A COMMUNITY TRUST
Nurse details are provided separately

2

JULY 1999 – SEPTEMBER 1999 INCLUSIVE
RNE version number 36

Figure 5.4 – Sample page from PACT catalogue.

- How do we marry prescribing data and caseload data to make meaningful comparisons between individual nurse prescribers, and to find 'outliers'?

- What arrangements does the trust have in place for identifying and dealing with prescribing indicative of poor practice?

Nurse prescribing within the context of clinical governance requires that all professionals who prescribe must be able to justify their treatment decisions. This means that nurses, doctors and pharmacists will have to sit down and talk together about prescribing. This offers a real opportunity to work together, pooling respective skills for the benefit of the people whose health needs we serve.

References

Department of Health (1999). *Review of Prescribing, Supply and Administration of Medicines* (Crown Report). London: Department of Health.

Department of Health (2000). *Health Services Circular* 2000/026 Patient Group Directions.

6

NURSE PRESCRIBING: AN EVALUATION OF AN IMPLEMENTATION PROGRAMME WITHIN ONE HEALTH AUTHORITY AND TWO COMMUNITY HEALTHCARE TRUSTS

The announcement by the Secretary of State for Health, at the Royal College of Nursing (RCN) annual conference in April 1998, that nurse prescribing would be extended in England ended 12 years of debate and expectancy. The implications of this announcement were that 20,000 qualified district nurses (DN) and health visitors (HV) would be funded centrally and that the implementation programme (Mode 1 training) would be achieved in three years.

The financial implications immediately became a major influencing factor. The funding, £550 per nurse, to meet education and training costs as well as the necessary support for implementation within practice would be available until the end of March 2001. Financial support for any DNs or HVs who did not achieve nurse-prescribing status during that period would not be met from a central fund but would rest with the individual nurse's employer. A further complicating factor is the projection that the community trusts concerned will be superseded by primary care trusts (PCTs) from April 2001. This innovation is likely to include changes in both the infrastructures and the personnel within the organisations.

At the same time, a nurse–prescribing element (Mode 2 students) would be added to the specialist community practitioner programmes for students taking the DN and HV specialist qualifying programmes. This would provide the normal route of education for new nurse prescribers and would become a requirement in order to gain the professional qualification which is recorded on the UKCC register for DNs and HVs.

In this chapter a case study will be presented which focuses upon the implementation process within one health authority (HA) and two adjoining community healthcare trusts which are located in one county. A critical analysis of the issues, which arose in relation to education and the implementation programme, will be presented. Finally, professional development needs will be discussed and concerns for the future noted.

THE EDUCATIONAL PROGRAMME

The issues that arose related to both the development and the evaluation of the course and included:

- accessing information
- developing relationships
- designing the course
- evaluating the programme.

Accessing information

The time limit imposed upon the central funding combined with the number of nurses who needed to qualify as prescribers were the two main factors that prompted the speed at which education programmes needed to be developed, validated by the English National Board for Nursing Midwifery and Health Visiting (ENB) and on offer to the community trusts. The two documents, *Nurse Prescribing: A Guide for Implementation* (NHSE, 1998) and *Recommendations for Nurse Prescribing Courses* (ENB,

1998, 1998a), were essential to the development of the nurse-prescribing course but were not distributed until late December 1998. Supplies of the *Nurse Prescribing Open Learning Pack* (ENB, 1998b), the Nurse Prescribers' Formulary (NPF) (BMA/RPS, 1998) and the ENB video were restricted to one of each per educational institution.

An added challenge was the market culture in which education was commissioned and the possible temptation for HAs to compromise on quality for the sake of economy. Educational institutions, on the other hand, may have been tempted to reduce fees inappropriately in order to secure the contract without due regard for the resource implications associated with the actual running of the course. In the case under review, the responsibility for choice of educational institutes was delegated to the community trusts.

A review of the literature which focused upon the nurse-prescribing pilot projects provided a valuable resource of information regarding the course content, teaching strategies, assessment procedures, overall evaluation of the course and the experience of nurse prescribers in practice (Luker *et al*, 1997; Blenkinsopp *et al*, 1998; Bentley and Leatham, 1998). A meeting with DNs and HVs who were employed by a neighbouring trust and who had been nurse prescribers since 1994 provided an opportunity to learn from their experience and to consider their views in relation to the length, content and delivery of the course.

Developing relationships

A relationship, established early in the implementation process, between the HA, both trusts and a representative from the educational institute enhanced collaboration in considering the issues that were immediately apparent in initiating the roll-out of nurse prescribing in the local setting. This did not, however, guarantee immediate, automatic education provider status. Outlines of nurse-prescribing course programmes were offered in the form of tenders to HAs in order to secure contracts to be nurse-prescribing educational providers. Evidence of one such contract was necessary before the ENB would consider validation for the course.

The educational institution on which this discussion is based were offered a contract to be their sole provider for nurse prescribing by one of the trusts and a contract to be a partial provider by the other trust. The decision of the latter trust reflected their normal practice in accessing DN and HV specialist community practitioner qualifying courses. This allowed students to make a choice and reduced the travelling for nurses who were based in the east of the county. Practice nurses with a DN or HV qualification who were employed by GPs but worked within the county were also allowed to choose which of the two educational programmes they preferred. The completion of these arrangements early in 1999 enabled a collaborative emphasis to be maintained and enhanced the speed and smooth running of the proposed developments.

Designing the course

A steering committee was established and regular meetings hosted by the health authority included the medical officer, community pharmacist and financial officers as well as nurse managers and course leaders. Occasional visits from the regional nurse for prescribing brought encouragement and the opportunity to learn from the experiences that related to a wider perspective.

Curriculum development meetings were juxtaposed with the steering group and consisted of DN and HV tutors, two nurses working as independent consultants, one with combined expert knowledge of applied anatomy and physiology and pharmacology and the second with expert legal knowledge and its application to nursing practice. A pharmacist and a GP joined the team prior to the commencement of the course. Discussions continued with nurse prescribers who had qualified within the pilot initiatives. They provided invaluable insights regarding the course and some of the issues that had arisen for them in practice. They agreed to facilitate a session within the course, which would focus particularly upon the practice implications that arise for nurse prescribers.

The ENB provided guidelines relating to the academic level, the aims and learning outcomes, the content, length of the course and the type of assessment to be used. All students received the open learning pack (ENB, 1998b) prior to commencing the course and the ENB video formed a bridge which enabled the student to integrate and build on this knowledge within the taught aspect of the course.

Assessment was in the form of an unseen examination. A broad outline for the structure of the examination paper, to include multiple choice or short answer questions and assessment and evaluation of two scenarios that reflect the real world of practice, was provided. The actual papers were developed independently by the individual education providers. This raised issues of uniformity in the academic level and the rigour implicit within these assessments. Although scrutiny and validation by the ENB education officers should provide assurance of equity, feedback at a recent ENB (1999) regional workshop suggested that this may not be the case. Particular issues of the percentage mark required to achieve a pass and regulations imposed regarding a second attempt were raised and evidence of wide variations in practice recorded.

The course design spreads over nine weeks (see Chapter 1) and includes a half-day introduction to the course which focuses upon:

- the open learning pack
- an introduction to anatomy and physiology for nurse prescribers
- setting up support networks
- dealing with concerns.

Two full days occur in week 5 and a third full day in week 6.

The course content builds upon the seven sections of the distance learning pack and includes:

- pharmacology and the NPF
- legal and ethical issues
- communication and assertiveness
- working in teams
- audit and evaluation
- budgets and administration
- clinical supervision
- implementing nurse prescribing in practice.

The final half-day in week 7 accommodates the examination. Students receive their examination results within two weeks and any students who do not pass are informed by telephone by the course tutor. They are offered tutorial support and an opportunity to undertake a further examination at a mutually convenient time.

An external examiner was appointed and the first Examination Board arranged on completion of the first programme and the following guidelines for examination procedure were agreed.

- Subsequent Examination Boards would be held at six-monthly intervals

- The External Examiner would moderate all examination questions

- A sample of all the students' examination papers to include all borderline or failed papers

- The Chair of the Examination Board would take action to confirm examination results, which occurred in the intervening time between the designated Examination Boards.

The first course, of a two-year programme, commenced on 31 March 1999 and it is expected that around 400 nurses will have completed the course and have prescribing status by March 2001.

Evaluating the programme

Evaluation has focused upon the following issues.

- The open learning pack
- Time
- Study skills
- Course content
- Assessment
- Administration.

The open learning pack

The open learning pack has been positively evaluated and found to fulfil its intended purpose in forming a foundation for the course programme, which follows. A positive attribute is the conceptual framework within which nurse prescribing is presented in the pack, which includes professional accountability, safe prescribing, legal issues, ethical issues, teamwork, administration and evaluation. A number of students have applied the concepts to their wider professional practice and found it to be an ideal evaluation tool.

Time

The four-week interval between the introduction and first full day of the course has provided a sufficient time lapse for the majority of practitioners to complete the pack. However, the scarcity of nurses and the increased pressures generated by constant changes within the healthcare system have for some practitioners compounded the difficulty in finding the required time for study within working hours. The official amount of study time allocated by both trusts is one day, to be taken to prepare for the examination. This has depended upon colleagues being willing to cover caseloads but has been accessed by the majority of DN and HV students.

The availability of time for practice nurses (PNs) has depended upon the attitude of their employers. Some GPs have welcomed the implementation of nurse prescribing and supported the nurses in accessing the course by allowing time for the necessary study. Others have not and in this case, nurses who work in single GP practices have been particularly disadvantaged. This problem has continued for PNs in the postqualifying period in relation to participation in learning sets and practice development workshops.

Study skills

The level of academic experience with which the students enter the course is an important determinant in relation to the amount of stress experienced. For those who have little experience of study in higher education and who gained their professional qualifications through certificate-level courses, the task appears daunting and the language is often unfamiliar. The formation of multidisciplinary study groups within reasonable geographical locations is encouraged at the introductory session. These enable students to share knowledge and resources, to maximise the use of time and provide support for one another. Community practice teachers and team leaders were encouraged to access the early nurse-prescribing courses and have acted as mentors to colleagues undertaking the course. However, it is anticipated that there may be a rise in the number of students needing extra support in the later courses. A six-hour study skills programme has been offered in an attempt to minimise the problem.

Course content

The Medicinal Products: Prescription by Nurses etc. Act 1992, which provided the legislation for some nurses to become independent prescribers, was of historical significance. It has, however, introduced nurses to a new sphere of legal accountability and in turn has highlighted the importance of the *Code of Professional Conduct* and the *Scope of Professional Practice*. Evaluation of the ethical and legal content of the course has been good and has demonstrated the value of considering nursing issues from a legal perspective as the accountability issues do not rest with nurse prescribing alone. Many students undertaking the nurse-prescribing course completed their qualifying courses many years ago and have not considered the importance of professional accountability in the increasingly litigious climate in which community nursing is practised today. There is potential for this new awareness to prompt further development and growth leading to improvement in patient care but also to act as a deterrent to possible falling standards in practice.

An up-to-date knowledge of the life sciences was deemed to be essential in order to complement the basic pharmacology knowledge required (While and Rees, 1993; Jordon and Potter, 1999). Problems for students in confidently recalling knowledge of the life sciences, which may have been studied very early in their professional education and training, were anticipated. A second open learning pack (Courtenay, 1999), which provides a revision programme focused upon the life sciences relevant to the current formulary, is given to each nurse at the introductory session. This can be updated and added to as required and maximises the use of time by providing instant access to the relevant information.

Most nurses have only a basic knowledge of pharmacology and it is therefore essential to address the whole formulary in the limited time available. Luker *et al* (1997) are critical of the limited NPF but as the formulary is extended so there will be implications for an increase in the associated amount of knowledge in both the life sciences and pharmacology.

Student-centred learning methods, including role play, have been used in order to focus upon communication, self-awareness and teamwork. The students have been encouraged to share incidents from their own practice experience and the use of problem-solving techniques is discussed. The balance of power between doctors and nurses within teams in general practice is often viewed negatively by nurses and the contribution of two GPs to the course has provided a forum to explore the possible implications for nurse prescribers.

Initially a DN and a HV from a neighbouring trust, who were part of the nurse-prescribing pilot project, provided a useful session. This focused upon issues from practice and demonstrated how they had worked successfully with GPs to prepare guidelines and solve any problems or differing perceptions they had in relation to the prescribing role. After six months the visiting DN and HV handed over to a similar partnership from within the local trusts. GP fundholding had been replaced by primary care groups (PCG) and many of the students' questions related to local issues. The value of the initial contribution was never doubted but the incorporation of local practitioners within the taught programme was gratifying in that it provided evidence of real progress in the implementation programme.

Tutors and practitioners have learned together as the experience of nurse prescribing evolves. The tensions felt by the tutors have moved from concerns regarding the design and delivery of the course to managing the considerable increase in administrative workload in maintaining the number of courses needed to complete the task in the allocated time. The students no longer feel that they are being used as 'guinea pigs'. However, the stress associated with the acquisition of new knowledge and the associated assessment remains.

Assessment

In order to qualify as a nurse prescriber, an unseen examination taken on day 5 of the course must be passed. This includes multi-choice and short answer questions which form part one of the written examination. Part two examines practice and consists of four practice-based scenarios. The student must choose two of the scenarios and for each, make an assessment and provide a critical evaluation, which demonstrates safe and effective practice in relation to nurse prescribing.

A pass at 70% for part one has not created problems but achieving a 50% pass level for part two, has been more difficult for some. The high level of tension generated by the examination itself does not enhance recall and clarity of thought. For the small minority who do not pass the examination at the first attempt, the embarrassment of being seen to be unsuccessful by their peers is the most sensitive issue. Attempts are always made to be supportive and discreet in communicating information of this nature and in setting up the resit opportunity. To date all have been successful at the second attempt.

Administration

The frequency of the courses has exacerbated the amount of administrative work involved. Good communication networks between the course leader, an able secretary and the nurse prescriber project nurses have been essential for the efficient running of the programme. The production of examination papers and a commitment to announce examination results within a two-week schedule has depended upon the continued co-operation of tutors with marking responsibilities and the External Examiner returning moderated work within a tight time framework. Facilitative skills have also been required in co-ordinating the needs of internal and visiting lecturers.

Only minimal reference can be made to the first cohort of DN and HV students currently undertaking the specialist community practitioner qualifying course (Mode 2 students). The main issues that are currently apparent for them are the added pressure of an examination in an already heavily assessed course and the inequity created by the fact that only two of seven specialist options that are represented within the student cohort are included. This is a significant problem to the PNs who feel strongly that they should be included.

THE IMPLEMENTATION PROGRAMME

Within the NHS Executive guidelines for the implementation of nurse prescribing (NHSE, 1998), there is a clear indication of the need to implement a strategy that is specific to the requirements of local HAs and trusts. In fact, the release of the NPF, the open learning pack and the National Prescribing Centre bulletins to HAs and trusts was dependent upon an implementation plan being submitted to the NHS Executive headquarters. This plan included an assessment of the number of nurses who would become nurse prescribers within the timescale allotted and the estimated cost.

The complexity of the issues that needed to be addressed was reflected in the membership of the groups that provided an infrastructure for the implementation of the strategy.

An advisory group was established at the HA early in 1999 with senior nurse representatives from each trust, the HA and the educational institutes as well as representatives from the local medical and pharmaceutical committees. The trusts also inaugurated multidisciplinary management teams consisting of a professional development nurse, a community pharmacist, a risk manager, a personnel manager, a finance manager and a GP.

Tasks to be addressed included:

- the appointment of project nurses
- the accessing and safe storage of prescription pads
- the standardisation of record keeping.

Project nurses

The trusts were influenced by the evaluation of the Walsall and Wigan pilot sites which acknowledged project management as a critical factor for the successful implementation of nurse prescribing (Blenkinsopp *et al*, 1998). As a result two project nurses, a HV in the east and a DN in the west, were appointed. Financial support was provided from the central nurse-prescribing funding.

The project nurses were early recruits to the nurse-prescribing course and after qualifying as nurse prescribers, they were adopted on to the advisory group and the trust management teams. They also facilitated a steering group of recently qualified nurse prescribers who reviewed decisions made by the management group in relation to their own practice experience. This produced a partnership approach between managers and practitioners, which aimed to develop and monitor a strategy which was effective in its purpose of implementing nurse prescribing.

The project nurses were seconded to the project for two days per week and were allocated administrative assistance. Their role demanded advanced skills in the following areas.

Management

Initially the role of the project nurses appeared to be functional in managing the uptake of nurses on to the available nurse-prescribing courses in order to ensure that all eligible nursing staff had completed their training by March 2001. The reality was in fact a more complex challenge and included skills in negotiation and integration in order to co-ordinate course dates with annual leave, other professional development needs of potential nurse prescribers as well as their colleagues' availability in maintaining a safe level of nursing and health-visiting care.

Teaching

As soon as they became confident in their nurse-prescribing role, they agreed to teach two sessions on the nurse-prescribing course. This fulfilled two functions: first, an opportunity to offer support to their peers and second, a convenient meeting place to collect and disseminate information. The first session was in the form of an introduction to nurse prescribing in practice and was scheduled on the introductory day. The second session was scheduled on day 4 of the course and addressed implications for practice, which had been raised during the course, and any trust developments that related specifically to nurse prescribing.

Support

A further demanding but essential task has been the support of practitioners whose insecurity and stress have led to expressions of frustration and anger.

Prescription pads

Three important issues specific to prescription pads are:

- safe delivery
- security
- guidelines and procedures.

Safe delivery

This was more eventful than anticipated. Placing the order with the Stationery Office proved to be straightforward but delivery of the pads was initially prolonged and included a postal tour of three southern counties before eventually arriving at their destination.

Security

The problem encountered above led the management team to abandon an original plan to have the prescription pads delivered to individual GP practices. Both of the trusts have a number of community hospitals that are geographically spread throughout the location. The pads are delivered to a specific department in each hospital where security can be maintained. The individual nurse prescribers collect their own prescription pads from this secure base. This solves the problem of limited storage space in some GP practices and also eradicates the need for a third person to be involved.

Guidelines and procedures

Guidelines and procedures concerning the entire process, from the original order of the prescription pad to its delivery, advice about the security and what to do if the pad is stolen, have been issued in two formats, one to each GP practice or health centre and an A5 version to each nurse. The latter can be carried within the practitioner's diary.

Record keeping

The standardisation of record keeping has been difficult to implement mainly because of the variety of systems used within the GP practices. Some retain handwritten records while others are totally computerised. It has been necessary to establish general principles and delegate the responsibility to individual nurse prescribers to negotiate with the GPs in their own practices regarding the recording of prescribed products.

EVALUATION OF THE IMPLEMENTATION PROGRAMME

Evaluating the implementation strategy has raised a number of significant issues, which will be considered under the following headings.

- Collaboration within the organisations
- Workforce issues
- The appointment of project nurses
- Practice issues.

Collaboration within the organisations

The collaboration between the advisory group, the management teams and the project nurses has proved to be an immensely positive experience. Nurse prescribing has been introduced with a sense of uniformity across the HA and within both community trusts. This has allowed problems to be addressed and examples of best practice to be shared. Some illustrations of ongoing work will be discussed in the final section and this is accompanied by an optimism that the scene may be set for a far wider agenda than nurse prescribing. This may be of significant importance in light of concerns that the shift from PCG/Ts to PCTs in April 2001 may result in the fragmentation of professional support networks.

Workforce issues

The projection, very early in the process, of the numbers of nurses who would become nurse prescribers in the allotted timescale has, with time for reflection, raised concerns. The movement of DNs and HVs in and out of the trusts, job shares and some seconded to other posts or courses as well as nurses returning through Back to Nursing courses may not have been considered in the original calculations. Some further funding may be required in order to meet their educational needs.

The introduction of nurse prescribing coincided with a shortfall in the number of nurses recruited generally and in particular, to meet the needs of community nursing services. A high percentage of DNs and HVs employed in both trusts could take retirement at any time. Although nurse prescribing has not been made a mandatory requirement for all practitioners in either of the trusts, there are concerns that the stress associated with its implementation may result in some people bringing forward their retirement date. Nurses accessing Return to Community Nursing courses may need particular consideration and require added support in their new role as prescriber. Also students undertaking the specialist community practitioner course in health visiting and district nursing will find themselves with an added assessment challenge in order to meet the qualifying requirements.

The project nurse

The appointment of the nurse-prescribing project nurses has had many benefits. The collaboration between trusts has already been mentioned but providing a named person with whom practitioners can communicate is of equal value. They are viewed as having empathy with the practitioners who are concerned by the stressful aspects of prescribing but also have enough influence to be able to deal with practice issues in an effective manner. However, for the project nurses themselves many issues have arisen. These have included the added stress of being offered the appointment prior to completing the qualifying course, the challenge of juggling a developing project role with the demands of managing their own caseload and maintaining good working relationships within their own community nursing teams. For one of the trusts, an unforeseen problem was the resignation of the project nurse. This unexpected situation may lead to reflection on the possible limitations of an initial, short-term secondment contract, which the trust were planning to extend.

Practice issues

Although guidelines and procedures relating to the security of prescription pads were developed early in the implementation period, an incident involving a stolen prescription pad highlighted a deficiency in the procedure. The nurse prescriber's diary was also stolen in which she had placed the guidelines outlining the actions to be taken if such a situation arose. In response to this incident, a copy of the guidelines is also included in DN and HV handbooks at each base.

Anomalies may occur in relation to what is taught within the course and the reality in practice. Legal accountability suggests that any product prescribed by a nurse for a patient is lawfully owned by the patient. Any acquisition of stock accumulated from unused patient products and stored in the boot of a nurse's car for emergency use amounts to fraud. The first Crown Report (DoH, 1989) recommended that nurses should be provided with a stock of products for emergency use by their employing agency. The number of changes that have occurred within the context in which primary healthcare is delivered may necessitate a review of this recommendation. There is a great deal of sensitivity in relation to prescribing budgets and concern that influential GP, PCG/T or PCT members may not be sympathetic to the provision of emergency stock for nurses unless clear guidelines are issued.

The anxiety experienced by nurse prescribers when writing their first prescriptions was highlighted by Luker *et al* (1998) and has also been acknowledged in the two trusts under review. The realisation of responsibility in signing the prescription, rather than passing it to the GP, is marked. This may reflect the emphasis within the course on the importance of professional and legal accountability. In order to rationalise this stress, nurse prescribers are encouraged to work with an established nurse prescriber, GP or pharmacist who will act as a mentor until confidence is gained. This form of collaboration in practice may enhance team working in general.

POSTQUALIFYING SUPPORT

Support in the postqualifying period is needed in relation to:

- nurse prescribers
- a substantive, lead nurse post
- financial strategies.

Nurse prescribers

Learning sets were initially set up in both trusts. These were facilitated by the project nurses and aimed to provide a forum in which issues relevant to practice could be addressed and support provided for new nurse prescribers. These were found to be beneficial by some but others were prevented from attending because of demanding caseloads or, in the case of practice nurses, no one to provide relief for clinics. Both the project nurses believed that appropriate training would have enhanced their role as facilitators.

Practice nurses are employed by the GPs and any corporate management is through the HA. As there is no lead post in the HA for nursing, they felt vulnerable. In an attempt to address this issue, a lead nurse prescriber for practice nursing has been appointed in each trust. It is envisaged that these nurses will be a voice for practice nurses as inevitable changes occur in the move from PCG/Ts to PCTs.

The National Prescribing Centre has instigated regional study days. Although they have been positively evaluated, attendance is limited to a minority and the role of the centre is not expected to persist beyond March 2001.

Further professional study which is specifically related to nurse prescribing is an inevitable consequence of the widening of professional practice boundaries and any increase in the number of products in the NPF. Two workshops have been organised by the educational institution in collaboration with the trusts, one focusing upon differential diagnosis (see Chapter 4) and a second upon further legal issues (see Chapter 2).

A substantive lead nurse post

The project nurse posts are related specifically to the implementation strategy and are supported by central funding. They will cease in their current form at the same time as the community trusts are devolved and PCTs take responsibility for the professional development programme for community nurses. It would appear to be imperative that a lead nurse is appointed who is able to take overall responsibility for postqualifying education and support for nurse prescribers. Responsibilities would include the setting up of peer support and guidance through clinical supervision as well as providing a pivotal point for the implementation of new procedures and overall collaboration within the PCTs.

Financial strategies

The transition from PCG/Ts to PCTs will produce changes in the way in which budgets are managed. The intervening period will require the pharmaceutical advisers, heads of finance, lead and project nurses for prescribing to work collaboratively to provide advice and information to establish robust frameworks and guidelines in order to facilitate an effective transition period and a successful financial strategy for the future.

CONCLUSION

The introduction of nurse prescribing has depended upon an effective implementation strategy as well as a supporting education programme. Many issues have been raised for managers, educationalists and practitioners. This chapter has focused upon the initial processes and evaluated the outcomes. One of the positive attributes has been the increased level of collaboration that has occurred between the HA and the two community trusts.

Achievements so far are minimal compared with those that will be required in the future. Managing the change from PCG/Ts to PCTs will be a major task to be followed by many further challenges as the scope for nurse prescribing is widened to incorporate the remaining specialist community practitioners, specialist nurses and eventually the nursing profession as a whole.

Acknowledgements

I would like to thank Catherine Blowers and Mary Mullix for their contribution to this chapter.

References

Bentley, H. & Leatham, J. (1998). Nurse prescribing: a critical evaluation of training. *Primary Health Care* 8(1): 26–30.

Blenkinsopp, A., Grime, J., Pollock, K., Boardman, H. (1998). *Nurse Prescribing Evaluation 1: The Initial Training Programme and Implementation.* Keele: Keele University.

British Medical Association/Royal Pharmaceutical Society of Great Britain in association with the Health Visitors' Association and Royal College of Nursing (1998). *Nurse Prescribers' Formulary.* Shaftesbury: Blackmore Press.

Courtenay, M. (1999). *Anatomy and Physiology for the Nurse Prescriber.* Reading: University of Reading.

Department of Health (1989). *Report of the Advisory Group on Nurse Prescribing* (Crown Report). London: Department of Health.

English National Board for Nursing, Midwifery and Health Visiting (1998b). *Nurse Prescribing Open Learning Pack.* Milton Keynes: Learning Materials Design.

English National Board for Nursing, Midwifery and Health Visiting (1999). Notes of the Nurse Prescribing Workshop, 2nd December. London: ENB.

Jordon S. & Potter, N. (1999). Biosciences on the margin. *Nursing Standard* 13(25).

Luker, K., Austin, L., Hogg, C. (1997). *Evaluation of Nurse Prescribing: Final Report and Executive Summary.* Liverpool: University of Liverpool.

Luker, K., Austin, L., Hogg, C., Ferguson, B., Smith, K. (1998). Nurse patient relationships: the context of nurse prescribing. Journal *of Advanced Nursing* 28 (2): 235–242.

National Health Service Executive (1998). *Nurse Prescribing: A Guide for Implementation.* London: Department of Health.

While, A. & Rees, K. (1993). The knowledge base of health visitors and district nurses regarding products in the proposed formulary for nurse prescription. *Journal of Advanced Nursing* 18: 1573–1577.

INDEX

accountability, 9–24, 34–37, 94

acharis oil, 44

administration of training courses, 95–96

advisory groups, implementation programme, 96

alcoholic solutions, head lice, 53

allergic contact dermatitis, 44, 45

almond oil, 65

ambulances, Cooper's traffic lights illustration, 28

antibiotics, boils, 60–61

antifungal preparations, 55

anxieties *see* stress

Aspergillus nigra, ear infection, 64

aspirin, moral responsibility example, 36–37

assessment (examinations), nurse-prescribing course, 6, 90–92, 95

Atkin, Richard (Baron), definition of duty of care, 13

atopic dermatitis, 42, 44, 45, 46–47

auriscopes, 64

Back to Nursing courses, nurses from, 100

bacteria
ear infection, 64
nappy rash, 55
skin carriage, 61

Bateman, R v (1925), 15

bath oil, 48

beer bottle, snail, 13

Birmingham Water Works, Blyth v (1856), definition of negligence, 12

Blenkinsopp, A., *et al.*, pilot studies, 3–4

Blyth v *Birmingham Water Works* (1856), definition of negligence, 12

body lice, 53

boils, 60–61

Bolam test, 14–15

Bolitho v *City and Hackney Health Authority* (1993), 14–15

Bolton, pilot scheme, 4

Bowen's disease, 42

breast-feeding, thrush, 62, 63

budgets, 40–41, 77
monitoring, 79

'bug buster' treatments, 52, 53

bulk purchase, 75–76

bulk-forming laxatives, 57

burrows, scabies, 49–50

cancer of skin, 48

Candida albicans
nappy rash, 54, 55
thrush, 61–63

car boot *see* stocks, surplus

carbaryl, 52, 53

carbuncles, 60, 61

carriage of bacteria, 61

cash limits, 78

causal responsibility, 36

cavernous sinus thrombosis prevention, 60

central funding, implementation programme, 87–88

chlorhexidine, 61

City and Hackney Health Authority, Bolitho v (1993), 14–15

clinical governance, 85

clinical supervision, 22

Code of professional conduct (UKCC), 13

colleges (educational institutes), contracts, 89–90

commercial pressures, 18, 82
communication with colleagues, 21, 40
community nurse managers, 70
community pharmacists, 68, 71
community setting *see* non-community
    settings
community trusts/services
    implementation programme, 87–104
    pharmacists, 69
competence, maintenance, 22
    see also training
compliance, 33–35
confidentiality, 29–31
consent, 20
    compliance and, 34
constipation, 55–58
    children, 58
Consumer Protection Act 1987, product
    liability, 19
contact dermatitis, 44, 45
contracts, educational institutes, 89–90
Cooper, D, traffic lights illustration,
    26–27, 28
cosmetics *vs* medicines, 41
cost effectiveness, information sources
    on, 40–41
cost of prescriptions, 31–33
crab lice, 53
creams *vs* ointments, 48
Crown Report 1989, 1–2
Crown Report 1999, 4
    definitions in, 72
Cumberledge Report 1986, 1
curriculum development, 90

definitions
    in Crown Report 1999, 72
    duty of care, 13
    negligence, 12
demonstration sites *see* pilot schemes
dependent prescribers, 4, 11, 12
diabetes mellitus
    bacteria, 61
    thrush, 62
diagnosis, 41
distance learning *see* Open Learning
    Pack (ENB); open learning pack
    (life sciences)

Dobson, Frank (Health Secretary), 4
Donoghue v *Stevenson* (1932), 13
drainage, boils, 60
dressings
    boils, 60
    bulk purchase, 75–76
    ethics examples, 28, 29
    see also stocks, surplus
drug information centres, 70
drug information sources, 70
    on cost effectiveness, 40–41
duplication, medical records, 17–18, 40
duty of care, 12–14
    potential breaches, 16–21

ear
    syringing, 65
    wax, 63–65
eardrum, 64
East Kent, pilot site, 82
eczema, 45–47
    atopic dermatitis, 42, 44, 45, 46–47
education *see* training
educational institutes, contracts, 89–90
electronic PACT data, 79
emergency stocks, 101
emollients
    management, 48
    as medicines, 41
employers, 20–21
enemas, 57–58
English National Board (ENB), 90
    see also Nurse Prescribers' Formulary
        (NPF); Open Learning Pack (ENB)
ePACT (electronic PACT data), 79
ethical issues, 25–38
    training course content on, 94
examination (physical), rashes, 44–45
examinations, nurse-prescribing course,
    6, 90–92, 95
expenditure
    funding of training, 87–88
    monitoring, 78–79
    see also budgets
expressed consent, 20

face, 'danger area', 60–61
faeces, impaction, 57

Farquharson, Lord Justice, on Bolam test, 14–15
faxing of prescription (confidentiality issue), 30–31
fibre (dietary), 57
financial means, clients, 32
fluid requirements, 56
formularies, development of, 77
fraud, surplus stock accumulation as, 101
Friern Barnet Hospital Management Committee, Bolam v (1957), 14
funding
  expenditure monitoring, 78–79
  training, 87–88
  see also budgets
fungal infections, 43 (Fig.), 44, 46 (Table), 47–48
  ear, 64
  scalp and nails, 49
  skin, 45
  steroid creams and, 44, 49
  see also Candida albicans

general practice
  PACT data, 79–82
  receptionists, confidentiality and, 31
general practitioners (GPs), 17
  communication with, 40
  in nurse-prescribing course, 94–95
  study time availability and, 93
group protocols *see* Patient Group Directions (group protocols)
guidelines
  development of, 77
  prescription pads, 99, 101
  vs rules, 26

head lice, 51–54
health authorities
  implementation programme, 87–104
  pharmaceutical advisers, 68–69, 71
  pharmaceutical industry and, 77
Health Services Circular 2000/026, 73
health visitors, 22
herbal remedies, head lice and, 53
Hewart, Lord Justice, on standards of care, 15
history-taking, rashes, 44

hospital stores, supply from, 78
Hunt, Philip (Health Secretary), quoted, 5
hygiene, threadworms, 59

ignorance, unavoidable, 36
immunosuppression
  scabies, 50
  thrush, 62
impaction, faecal, 57
implementation programme, 87–104
  evaluation, 99–101
implied consent, 20
incapacity, moral responsibility and, 36–37
incision, boils, 60
independent prescribers, 4, 11, 12
information to patients
  product liability and, 19
  see also consent
insecticides
  head lice, 53
  scabies, 50
Internet, drug information, 70
'issue' (use of word), 25
itchy rashes, 44, 48–49

Kent (East), pilot site, 82

lactulose, 57
lancing, of boils, 60
lanolin, 44
law *see* legal framework for nurse prescribing
laxatives, 57
lead nurse posts, 102–103
learner drivers, accountability example, 10
learning methods
  student-centred, 94
  see also study skills
learning sets, 102
legal framework for nurse prescribing, training course content on, 94
lice, 51–54
lichenification, 45
life sciences, education on, 94
lindane, 53

macules, 42
magnesium sulphate paste, 60
malathion, 50, 53
managers, 20–21
   see also nurse managers; team managers
market culture (NHS), 89
means (financial), 32
mebendazole, 58
medical records, multiplicity, 17–18, 40
Medicinal Products: Prescription by
   Nurses etc. Act 1992, 2, 5, 11–12
(Commencement No 1) Order, 11
Medicines Act 1968, 10
medicines information centres, 70
medicines *vs* cosmetics, 41
mentoring, 101
miconazole gel, 63
microscopy, fungal skin infections, 48
money, ethics and, 31–33
monitoring, expenditure, 78–79
moral responsibility, 36–37
multidisciplinary management teams,
   implementation programme, 96–97
mycosis fungoides, 42

nails, ringworm, 49
nappy rash, 54–55
Naseptin, 61
National Institute of Clinical
   Effectiveness (NICE), 17
   cost effectiveness data, 41
National Prescribing Centre
   study days, 102
   website, 70
negligence, 12–16
Neighbourhood nursing (Cumberledge
   Report 1986), 1
neighbours, duty of care of, 13
Nettleship v *Weston* (1971), 10
New Prescribers Advisory Committee,
   4, 11–12
NHS trusts *see* trusts
NICE *see* National Institute of Clinical
   Effectiveness (NICE)
nipples, thrush, 62, 63
nits, 52
non-community settings, exclusion in
   legislation, 11

non-maleficence, 26
Norwegian scabies, 50
nose, bacteria carriage, 61
NPF *see* Nurse Prescribers' Formulary
   (NPF)
nurse managers
   community nurse managers, 70
   monitoring of prescribing, 79
nurse prescribers (Crown report 1999
   definition), 72
Nurse Prescribers' Formulary (NPF), 3,
   11
GPs prescribing items from, 79–82
nurse prescribing
   advantages and disadvantages, 73–74
   course (Mode 1 students), 6
   see also Open Learning Pack (ENB)
*Nurse prescribing: a guide for
   implementation*, 88–89
nurse specialists, 71
nurses, requests for prescriptions, 20–21
Nystatin, 63

ointments *vs* creams, 48
olive oil, 65
onychomycosis, 49
Open Learning Pack (ENB), 6
   distribution, 89
   evaluation of, 92
   on responsibility, 35
open learning pack (life sciences), 94
Orders (legislative), 11
OTC *see* over-the-counter (OTC)
   products
overspending, 78, 82
over-the-counter (OTC) products
accountability and, 17
ear wax, 65
vs prescribed treatments, cost issues, 32

PACT *see* Prescription Analysis and Cost
   Trends
papules, 42
Patient Group Directions (group
   protocols), 5, 72–75
   report on medicines supply under
   (1998), 4

patients
information for, product liability, 19
preference for nurse prescribing, 2–3
patient-specific written directions, 72–73
PCG, PCT *see* primary care groups,
trusts
peanut oil, 44
pediculosis, 51–54
peer support, 22
Pennells, E., on standards of care, 15
permethrin, 50, 53
personal development plans, 13–14
personal identification numbers,
prescription pads, 18–19
PGDs *see* Patient Group Directions
(group protocols)
pharmaceutical industry, 76–77
product literature, 70–71
see also commercial pressures
Pharmaceutical Services Regulations 1994,
10
pharmacists, 40, 67–71
pharmacology, education on, 94
pharmacy, 67–85
phenothrin, 53
pilot schemes, 2–4
input to training programme, 89,
94–95
PIN (personal identification numbers),
prescription pads, 18–19
piperazine (in Pripsen), 58
postqualifying support, 102–103
practice nurses
representation, 102
study time availability, 93
preferential prescribing, 18
Prescription Analysis and Cost Trends
(PACT)
reports and catalogues, 78–79, 83
(Fig.), 84 (Fig.)
for self-monitoring, 4
prescription pads
implementation programme and,
98–99
security, 18–19, 98–99, 101
prescriptions
cost, 31–33
writing, 16–18

primary care groups, trusts, 40, 41,
82–85, 88
group-to-trust transition, 103
pharmaceutical advisers, 69–70, 71
postqualifying support, 102–103
principles, 26–28
Pripsen, 58
product liability, 19
project nurses, 97, 100–101, 102–103
promotional literature, 18, 71
protocols, 26
psoriasis, 43 (Fig.), 45, 46 (Table)
psychosomatic symptoms, lice and, 51

qualifications of nurse prescribers, 5, 11
examinations, 6, 90–92, 95

R v *Bateman* (1925), 15
rashes, 42–55
receptionists, confidentiality and, 31
*Recommendations for nurse prescribing
courses*, 88–89
record keeping, 17–18, 40
implementation programme, 99
referrals
to colleagues, 41–42
constipation, clinical features
requiring, 56
regional study days, 102
responsibility, 34–37
see also accountability
Return to Community Nursing courses,
nurses from, 100
*Review of prescribing, supply and
administration of medicines report*
(1999), 11–12
ringworm *see* fungal infections
Rogers v *Whitaker* (1992), 14–15
role responsibility, 35–36
rules, 26–29
runs, scabies, 49–50

sales promotional literature, 18, 71
see also pharmaceutical industry,
product literature
scabies, 44–45, 46 (Table), 49–51
contact dermatitis from treatment, 44

scalp
    lice, 51–54
    ringworm, 49
scaly rashes, 45, 48–49
schools, lice outbreaks, 51
Scope of professional practice (UKCC), 22
    limits of knowledge and skill, 13
    vs Medicinal Products: Prescription by
        Nurses etc. Act 1992
        (Commencement No 1)
        Order, 11
    reflection on practice, 9
scratching, lichenification, 45
seborrhoeic dermatitis, 45, 46 (Table), 47
security, prescription pads, 18–19, 98–99,
    101
Sellotape, threadworms, 58
senna (in Pripsen), 58
shampoos (insecticidal), 53
Simanowitz, A., on Bolam test, 14
skin
    bacteria carriage, 61
    cancer, 48
    rashes, 42–55
snail in beer bottle (case), 13
solar keratoses, 42
South Thames Drug Information
    Centre, website, 70
specialist community practitioner
    programmes, 88
specialist nurses, 71
standards of care, 14–15
Staphylococcus aureus, 61
Stauch, M., on Bolam test, 14–15
steroid creams, 49
fungal infections and, 44, 49
steroid inhalers, thrush, 62
Stevenson, Donoghue v (1932), 13
stocks
    emergency, 101
    surplus, 26, 27–28
        legal implications, 101
stress
    examinations, 6, 90–92, 95
    writing first prescriptions, 3, 101
student-centred learning methods, 94
study days, regional, 102
study skills, 93

see also learning methods
study time, for Open Learning Pack, 93
sun exposure, 42
supervision, clinical, 22
suppositories, laxative, 57–58
surplus stocks *see* stocks, surplus
syringing, ear, 65

tea tree oil, head lice and, 53
team managers, ethics example, 29
tenders for contracts, educational
    institutions, 89
threadworms, 58–60
thrush, 61–63
time (study time for Open Learning
    Pack), 93
Tingle, J., on accountability, 13
toiletries *vs* medicines, 41
Touche Ross study 1991, 2
traffic lights illustration (Cooper), 26–27,
    28
training, 5–6, 7
    evaluation of, 92–96
    funding, 87–88
    implementation programme, 87–96
    maintenance of competence, 22
trusts
    PACT data, 79
    see also community trusts/services,
        pharmacists
tutors, 95
tympanic membrane, 64

UKCC *see* United Kingdom Central
    Council
underspending, 78, 82
unique nurse identifiers, prescription
    pads, 18–19
United Kingdom Central Council
    Code of professional conduct, 13
    disciplinary action, 15
    Scope of professional practice, 9

values, delimiting ethics, 25–26
vasectomy (case), failure of 'Bolam'
    defence, 14
venous eczema, 45
vicarious liability, 20–21

Walsall, pilot site, 3–4
waste, and costs, 33
websites, drug information, 70
Whitaker, Rogers v (1992), 14–15

Wigan, pilot site, 3–4
workforce, implementation programme, 100
workshops, postqualifying support, 102

NOTES

NOTES

NOTES

NOTES

NOTES

NOTES

NOTES